Madness and Murder

PETER MORRALL

PhD, MSc, BA(Hons), PGCE, RGN, RMN, RNMH

Senior Lecturer in Health and Sociology
University of Leeds

W
WHURR PUBLISHERS
LONDON AND PHILADELPHIA

© 2000 Whurr Publishers
First published 2000 by
Whurr Publishers Ltd
19b Compton Terrace, London N1 2UN, England and
325 Chestnut Street, Philadelphia PA 1906, USA

British Library Cataloguing in Publication Data
A catalogue record for this book is available from the British
Library.

ISBN: 1 86156 164 4

Contents

Preface

The theoretical approach I have adopted in this book owes much to the version of 'realism' devised by (among others) Professor Jock Young of Middlesex University. The following anecdote may have become embellished with the passage of time, or could even be apocryphal. However, I seem to recall that it was the now-renowned criminologist Jock Young who both dumbfounded and impressed a group of unrefined left-wing idealists (including myself) undertaking a sociology degree at a London polytechnic in the early 1980s. Speaking as a guest lecturer, he destroyed our simplistic but fervently held doctrine that most, if not all, criminal activity was the consequence of capitalist exploitation and materialism.

Our naive interpretation of the populist *Communist Manifesto* (which all of us had read) and impenetrable *Das Kapital* (which none of us had read) led us to assume that whilst every society had a persistent and irredeemable lumpenproletariat (criminal subclass), 'come the revolution' inequalities would disappear and crime figures would collapse. The 'new order' would mean that no-one would have any reason to steal as greed and avarice would have negligible meaning in a social system whereby each was given according to her or his need.

What Jock Young pointed out to us was that Marxists needed to accept and deal with the presence of crime, and recognize that much criminal activity (particularly muggings and burglary) was actually directed at the proletariat. Therefore, working-class people must, so the argument continued, defend themselves against nefarious elements in society. The social flaws of poverty and unemployment, generated by the capitalist mode of production, may be responsible for (some) crime, but this is not an adequate explanation of — or an excuse for — criminality.

The corollary of this realist perspective from the study of criminal behaviour, when applied to the subject of psychological disturbance, is that although constructed in various forms, there is an 'essentiality' to the category of madness. That is, to all intents and purposes, both badness and madness exist, and therefore have to be 'taken seriously'.

'You're mad!' said Zamyotov.....for some unknown reason, almost in a whisper, and again, for some unknown reason, he moved away suddenly from Raskolnikov. (Fyodor Mikhailovich Dostoyevsky, *Crime and Punishment*, 1866)

Introduction

Murder is the most malevolent of acts in a lengthy inventory of barbaric behaviours inaugurated by humans. Not only does the slaying of a man, woman or child destroy a life, but it also ravages the lives of all those associated with the person who has been killed, and foments the collective Angst of the community.

But the mad who kill are placed in a different socio-legal category from that of 'normal' murderers. Those regarded as insane, either at the time of their improbity or after the event, are propelled into a distinct and discreditable stratum of deviancy. They are 'unreasonably' dangerous. These miscreants are construed as 'double trouble' — mad and bad!

The consequence of entering the lowest end of the deviancy spectrum (only those convicted of child abuse lying further down the scale) can be drastic. Far longer periods of incarceration and greater quantities of social deformation are dispensed for a 'mad murder' than for an equivalent act that is perceived to be 'intelligible'.

However, only a small number of psychologically disturbed people are a danger to others. Individuals diagnosed as schizophrenic are much more likely to commit suicide than murder. The number of homicides carried out by 'normal' people is growing, whereas the homicide rate amongst the mentally disordered is relatively static. Why, therefore, was there at the end of the twentieth century such outrage concerning the mad murderer? Does this outrage represent yet another media-orchestrated 'panic' directed, as on previous occasions, towards an already marginalized and denigrated group? That is, are headlines like the following merely manifestations of a process in which a particular section of society,

considered a hazard to social stability, is demonized and scapegoated, thereby being neutralized?:

DANGER MENTAL PATIENTS EVADE CARE:
Public safety is being put at risk by more than 5,000 severely mentally ill
people who are being inadequately cared for in the community... .(Nicki
Pope, *Sunday Times*, 20 April 1997)

Alternatively, is there justifiable (if exaggerated) anxiety about
dangerous mentally disordered people being 'loose' in the community? Is there a genuine need to protect both society at large and the
mad? Does public concern over the homicidal tendencies of the
mentally disordered warrant emphatic social intervention to protect
both potential victims and perpetrators? What are the merits and
consequences of post-liberal mental health policies and laws, introduced at the end of the twentieth century and the beginning of the
twenty-first century in response to a declared failure of previous
approaches to the care of mentally disordered people and the protection of the public? How have the psychiatric disciplines of medicine
and nursing contributed to a period of unprecedented public alarm
in the 1990s with respect to the mentally disordered? These questions are addressed in this book.

The specific aim of the book is to evaluate critically, using
social science theory and empirical research findings, the incidents
of homicides perpetrated by people deemed to suffer from a
mental malfunction. Whereas there is a concentration on events in
Britain, the theories and research presented here have world-wide
applicability, although they are especially relevant to countries with
similar patterns of murder, and media, public and professional
reactions to homicide by the mentally disordered. Such countries
include the USA, Australia, New Zealand, South Africa and most
of Europe.

The target of my critique is the psychiatric disciplines of medicine and nursing. Members of these occupations are the most powerful (medicine) and numerous (nursing) in the field of mental health,
and have been the most vociferous in the 'defence' of practices that
have been given prominence in, and castigated by, the press. They,
out of all of those occupations that are employed in the 'psychiatric
industry' (the others principally being social workers, clinical

psychologists and occupational therapists), have been at the forefront of a campaign to 'dismiss' the problem of violence by their clients.

But it is the mental health disciplines of psychiatry and nursing as a totality, rather than any individual doctor or nurse, to which I am referring in this book. More specifically, this book is a polemic against the unified voice of conservative and progressive viewpoints within the mental health industry that arose over Madness and Murder. The mental health industry contains a disparate group of leaders, managers, practitioners and academics, who would normally disagree over all other issues, whether related to funda- mental precepts or everyday practices. In the 1990s, however, repre- sentatives of the 'mad business' formed an entrenched and expedient position, blaming the media for scaring the general population. I have depicted this confederated standpoint as that of the 'psychiatric establishment'.

In the first chapter, there is a necessary exposition of the core concepts underpinning the subject of Madness and Murder. Here 'crime' and 'insanity' are discussed. Specifically, the definitional and epistemological problems associated with these categories are high- lighted. Historical and contemporary policy trends concerning the mentally disordered are also examined. This then leads in Chapter 2 to a review of the conceptual and legal conjunctions between 'madness' and 'badness'. Here there is a tracing of the background to present legal interpretations of mental disorder for the purposes of court decisions on culpability. In Chapter 3, the issue of 'killing people' is explored. This includes discussions on the different forms of legal and unlawful killing, international rates of homicide and the incidence of murder committed by mentally disordered people.

The next four chapters contain theories that have attempted to enucleate the meaning and cause of both crime (including homicide) and the deviant category of mental disorder. In the first three of these chapters, the foremost explanatory genres in the field of criminology and deviancy are explicated. First, in Chapter 4, there is an exami- nation of those perspectives which characterize criminality and madness as abnormalities of the individual. These emanate in the main from reductionist, modernist and positivist conceptions of humanity. Here criminal and deviant behaviour is viewed either as the result of rational intent, or as being determined by psychological, evolutionary and biogenetic impulses. Within the explanatory genre, the endeavour of science is hypothesized as offering the prospect of a decline in or even elimination of many, if not all, forms of deviancy.

Social-causation approaches are tackled in Chapter 5. Within this explanatory framework, there is seen to be a correlation between crime and mental disorder and the way in which society is organized (or disorganized). Many of the perspectives that regard the structures and strains in the social system as having a direct influence on rates of crime and mental disorder are also reductionist, modernist and positivistic at their root. Just as psychological and biological conjecture on the 'faulty individual' leads to the notion of a 'cure', so the search for political, economic, cultural and ecological defects leads to a promise that through the scientific manipulation of the social (and/or physical) environment, the diminution of deviance is possible. The precepts of natural science are recruited into social science to correct the 'faulty society'.

The focus of Chapter 6 is on theories that are — in one way or another — the progeny of, or have made a contribution to, constructionist (or 'constructivist') accounts of the social and physical world. The extreme position of this theoretical camp is to view knowledge, reality and truth (and therefore crime and madness) as manufactured products of particular social groups, cultures or historical epochs. To be a criminal, or to experience madness, is, therefore, viewed as determined by the way in which those with power in society and/or the media implant 'faulty imagery'.

In consideration of the weaknesses of these three core theoretical frameworks that concentrate on redesigning the individual, on social insurrection or on readjusting the reaction of society to criminality and deviance, the paradigm of realism is presented *en rapprochement* in Chapter 7. Realism accepts that there is an underlying universal reality, although this is virtually impossible to 'know' accurately as it is always mediated through cultural forms. The experience of crime and mental disorder is, however, regarded as 'real enough', especially to the victims. This is no more so than when someone is killed. Hence, the realist perspective is critical of both positivist and constructionist explanations. Realism argues for the inclusion of the offender, the public, the state and the victim in the analysis of deviancy and crime.

The reality of the 1990s' 'terror' about 'mad killers' living in the community is appraised in Chapter 8. Data are presented from a 5-year study of media representations of homicides and non-fatal violence conducted by people described as mentally disturbed. Thousands of newspaper articles were reviewed, the content of which was contrasted with the 'facts' furnished by reports of independent inquiries into murders and other grievous incidents involving the mentally disordered.

Contrary to much of the extant literature on the handling of 'madness' by the press, and the stance taken by most mental health professionals, I conclude that homicide (whether by the 'mad' or 'normals') is a public health issue that should be taken not only seriously, but also whose rate has the potential to be checked. Moreover, the perceived dangerousness of the mentally disordered is 'realistic'. The threat to strangers and to the families and associates of the mentally disordered must be addressed by the psychiatric disciplines to prevent further persecution and scapegoating. When psychiatrists and nurses refuse to acknowledge their role as agents of social control, or the 'reality' of the danger posed by a limited number of their patients, they fuel public resentment and media panic.

Chapter 1
Crime and insanity

Deciding exactly what is and what is not a crime, and who is and who is not a criminal, is immensely complicated. These difficulties of definition are replicated when attempting to understand madness. In this chapter, I review some of the prevailing problems associated with rendering precise meanings for these categories of human behaviour.

This review centres on whether or not crime and madness can be regarded as objective facts that pervade all societies and are susceptible to accurate measurement and effective policies. Alternatively, do apparent variations in form across time, place and persons, as well as the routine appearance of impotent and chaotic policies, indicate that we cannot be secure in our knowledge of crime or madness, and that crime and madness are subjective and culturally relative concepts?

Criminality

A primary obstacle to fully comprehending crime and criminals is that of obfuscation. The concepts and propositions emerging from the discipline of criminology have come under severe attack for being vague and inconsistent (Gibbons, 1994). Moreover, the criminological body of knowledge itself is not united in its philosophical, epistemological and ontological appreciation of human conduct or of the nature and causes of transgressive behaviour. In particular, there is an historical disjunction between criminological and deviancy theories. This has its roots in the development of criminology, as a field of study, along 'modernist' principles, and the eventual

contraposition adopted by those who regard 'crime' not as an unam-
biguous category but as a manifestation of specific social processes.

Although modernism has its antecedents in the ancient world,
the Enlightenment exemplified a distinctive 'age of reason' during
the eighteenth century. The Enlightenment movement was built
upon the rationalist beliefs of Pascal, Locke, Newton and Descartes,
and the emancipatory entreaties of Hume, Diderot, Kant, Voltaire
and Rousseau. Progressive ideas about the freedom of the individual
and rationalism vied with religion and superstition to explain the
natural world. Science, technology and education were to provide
'logical' answers to the problems of the physical environment. Society was construed as being in a state of perpetual advancement
towards a better future, and the individual was adorned not only
with rights, but also with the responsibility for his or her own actions
and destiny.

These sociopolitical precepts of rationalism and individualism
were to furnish immense changes in the economic sphere: the
demise of feudalism, the expansion of industrialisation and the
ascent of the capitalist mode of production. Under these conditions,
the legal system (representing the values of the capitalist state) is
portrayed as upholding justice and truth, and perceptions of criminality are viewed as arising from individual pathology and malefac-
tion. Consequently, crime is regarded as innately iniquitous and is
defined narrowly as the infringement of an unimpeachable legisla-
ture. From this 'essentialist' approach, crimes are:

> wrong *not* because they violate a given society's or group's norms, rules, or
> laws, but because they are *objectively* wrong or *absolutely* evil. (Goode, 1996,
> p7, original emphasis)

However, by the twentieth century, the emerging social sciences
were challenging the notion of personal culpability as the only
explanatory factor that needed to be considered when looking for
the roots of human action. This has particularly been the contribution of the branch of sociology that acknowledges the determining
effect of society and its structures on behaviour. When applied to
crime, social-deterministic perspectives argue that organizational
and cultural settings must be taken into account when attempting to
understand criminality and decide upon punishment. From this

perspective, the violation of the law is an inadequate interpretation of crime: the criminal is seen as having broken wider and mutable social norms.

However, although a number of sociological approaches discussed later (for example, social disorganization and social strain theories) have incorporated the effects of social structures and processes into their exegesis of crime, they are still essentialistic and aetiological at heart. That is, there remains at the centre of their analysis an acceptance of a knowable and codifiable act committed by an identifiable individual or group. The basic question for these theorists, in common with causative interpretations coming from biology and psychology, is 'Why is this person (or why are these people) committing criminal acts?' More specifically, these theorists are asking, 'What is it about the biological make-up, psychological characteristics or the social milieu that leads to this person's criminal behaviour?'

Other sociological theories, however, go much further by questioning the whole enterprise of crime. Here a radically different definition of crime, and set of questions about the properties of criminality, are produced. Crime is not adjudged to be a consistent, tangible and circumscribed activity. Criminals are redefined as 'deviants' and are seen to be victims of the prejudices and self-interested defining of particular (usually powerful) groups in society:

> deviance is subjective rather than objective, relative rather than absolute, constructed rather than essentialistic. What deviance *is* does not depend on the inner, intrinsic, or inherent properties an act ... might have – that is its objective characteristics. Instead, what makes an act deviant is what certain people (or audiences) make of that act – what they think of it and how they react to it. (Goode, 1996, p8, original emphasis)

Consequently, acts of crime in one society may not have been construed as such in previous eras or may not be so considered in the future. Moreover, there will be little commonality across nations in the nature and incidence of crime.

However, the degree to which cultural and temporal variations affect the manufacture and constitution of crime has been contested. For example, Gottfredson & Hirschi (1990) postulate that consistencies in all societies between types of crime and the characteristics of the offender (for example, young men being responsible for most incidents of violent crime) indicate that different cultural contexts merely alter the opportunities available to commit crime. Gottfredson and Hirschi's project is to formulate a general theory of all crime. In doing so, they adopt a definition of crime ('acts of force or fraud undertaken in pursuit of self interest': 1990, pp172–3) that can be applied universally only because it is in itself so general.

What can, however, be seen to be universal is the centrality of 'control' over activities that may undermine the stability of society. The issue of 'social control' is embodied within the assemblage of theories that focus on the construction of deviant categories, but is also indirectly and implicitly an underlying premise of all criminology theory. Crimes and deviancies are social aggravations that involve either immediate or latent regulation by the state or its affiliated institutions of subjugation. Legal, political, religious, educational and medical institutions all assist in the preservation of 'acceptable' forms of behaviour and in the maintenance of a stable social system.

Every form of human society indulges in measures of social regulation. Without 'order', in its broadest sense, there would be no society:

> It is a truism that all societies, including the most unjust, unequal, disorganized and anomic ones, manifest certain structured patterns of interaction and routine behaviour which we refer to in aggregate as 'social order'. Otherwise we would not call them societies. (Scheerer & Hess, 1997, p105)

Threats to either the whole fabric of the social system, or to the people who have gained prestige, power and wealth within that system, are mollified by the organizations of social control. Social systems are liable to internal change, for example as a result of alterations in the status and influence of various groups. Moreover, external pressures, as a consequence, for example, of the globalization of technologies and economies, may cause prolonged periods of turmoil in the cultural practices of a society. The foundations of most societies are, however, intrinsically adaptable and durable. The structural fabric of society is only at risk of total disintegration when facing extraordinary circumstances such as civil war, invasion by a foreign power or economic collapse.

Not only do social control measures protect society as a whole, but the insecurities of the individual, generated by the predicaments (ethical and otherwise) of everyday existence, are also assuaged. Anthony Giddens (1991) suggests that there has in the industrialized world been a 'sequestration' of unsettling experiences, including those of 'nature', death, sickness, sexuality, criminality and madness:

> the ontological security which modernity has purchased, on the level of day-to-day routines, depends on an institutional exclusion of social from fundamental existential issues which raise central moral dilemmas for human beings. (Giddens, 1991, p156)

That is, the modern state and its institutions of control attempt to lessen its citizens' feelings of vulnerability and thereby evade primary questions on the meaning of life that may spawn new ideologies and insurrection. With various degrees of success, the physical environment is tamed, the dying removed from public view, the sick regulated and eroticism confined to the bedroom. Moreover, social deviants are stigmatized and/or interned, and the mentally disordered are medicalized and kept under supervision.

Coercion by the authorized agencies of social control is substantially reinforced by a complex series of informal networks that emerge from shared values (Mathews, 1993). We are constantly bombarded with both overt and subliminal signs from significant others. These signs shape the ways in which we perform as social beings by either encouraging or inhibiting our behaviour. Informal sanctions include mockery, reprimands, praise and an array of non-verbal communication such as frowns, smiles, touch and violent blows. We are, therefore, socialized into adopting the dominant convictions and socially approved patterns of behaviour through fear of condemnation by social control agencies and the media, as well as by affirmative and confrontative messages from members of our family, friends and peers.

For Mathews (1993), understanding the effectiveness of these informal mechanisms of social control leads to the realization that a reduction in the level of certain categories of crime (for example, burglary) can be achieved through local initiatives such as 'neighbourhood watch' schemes. Furthermore, the permeation of power into a multitude of social institutions other than those under the immediate and day-to-day subjugation of the state has resulted in the control of some forms of deviant behaviour being devolved to the point at which human interaction takes place. For example, the 'relatively autonomous' profession of medicine has licit powers to detain and, in certain circumstances, forcibly administer treatment to those deemed to be 'mad'. Psychiatric nurses also exercise control. This occurs in part through collaborating with medicine in its overt regulatory procedures, but mostly through persuasive mechanisms that ensue as a consequence of the 'therapeutic relationship' developed between the nurse and the psychiatric patient.

An understanding of the pervasiveness and effectiveness of social control does not, however, necessarily need to lead to the conclusion that all manifestations of the exercise of restraint are negative or only in the interests of a powerful élite. The legitimized defining and policing of criminality ensures not only that behaviour harmful to both the individual (physically or financially) and society (in terms of stability) is tempered, but also that the welfare of the deviant is monitored and protected. As Cockerham (1996) has pointed out, the alternative to social control, especially where 'dangerousness' is concerned, is disorder and the likelihood of human rights abuses of large sections of the population. Notwithstanding the unfortunate incidents of false imprisonment, and the need to confront inequity, the absence of potent and widespread control mechanisms would result in anarchy, social disintegration and barbarism.

More devastatingly, however, for the adherents of scientific rationalism and essentialism has been the iconoclastic philosophizing of postmodernist writers. Within the postmodern critique lies the proposition that all knowledge is uncertain. For postmodernist thinkers, the world in the late twentieth century has been going through a series of tumultuous transformations. Established social systems have had to react to a reordering of previous economic arrangements between societies, the creation of globalized markets and communication systems, the death of the 'expert' as the purveyor of absolute truth, and a metamorphosis in cultural values:

> we may no longer be living under the aegis of an industrial or capitalist culture which can tell us what is true, right and beautiful, and also what our place is in the grand scheme, but under a chaotic, mass-mediated, individual-preference-based culture of postmodernism. (Waters, 1994, p206)

From this outlook, there is no *a priori* moral, political or legal authority available to judge individual and social behaviour. All conduct (including deviancy) thus becomes relative to the particular practices of the social group to which individuals belong. Definitions of crime change over time and between cultures. Cannabis can be consumed legally in some countries, whereas in other countries a heavy fine or even imprisonment is imposed for its use. But even in parts of the world where using cannabis has been criminalized, it (along with derivatives of other prohibited drugs such as heroin) may be prescribed for medical purposes.

There are not just inconsistencies in what is determined to be a crime, but also tremendous variations in how crimes are dealt with. Whereas murderers in many parts of the USA may be executed, in Western Europe a gaol sentence will be handed out. In the People's Republic of China, the death penalty is given for a range of criminal activities other than murder (for example, drug dealing and political agitation). The Jordanian penal code allows a man to kill, without any penalty, his wife or a female relative if she is discovered committing adultery. Furthermore, political pragmatism and/or alterations in public opinion may dramatically affect punishment. For example, following the implementation of Section 2 of the 1997 Crime (Sentences) Act in England and Wales, there is now a mandatory life-sentence for a second violent or sexual offence. These second offences include attempted murder, manslaughter, soliciting murder, possession of a firearm with intent to injure, wounding or causing grievous bodily harm with intent, possession of a real or imitation firearm during a robbery, rape or attempted rape, and intercourse with a girl under 13 years of age. It is commonplace for punishments to be adjusted following the disclosure of an offender's previous criminal conviction(s). What is different here, however, is that, for a disparate and subjectively selected assemblage of crimes, there is minimal opportunity for a judge to do anything but give a predetermined sentence.

Furthermore, the criminal justice system casts its net of prohibition over a huge and multivaried list of activities (from not paying a television licence, riding a bicycle on the pavement and the underage drinking of alcohol, to grand larceny, grievous bodily harm and murder). It also operates a dual system of culpability based on the responsibility of the individual for his or her crime and the need to safeguard the community and social order:

> In English Law, for example, some offences such as murder, theft or serious assaults are described as *mala in se* or wrong in themselves. These are often seen as 'real crimes' in contrast to acts which are *mala prohibita*, prohibited not because they are morally wrong but for the protection of the public. (Croall, 1998, p4)

Moreover, there is also a wide disparity between what counts as the official crime rate, as recorded by the police, and the prevalence of crime. For example, the British Crime Survey (BCS) is a more comprehensive measure of legal infractions as it includes crimes not reported to the police. The method of investigation used in the BCS involves interviewing a representative sample of the population (who live in private households) to ascertain the experience of crime as described by its victims. Findings from the BCS indicate that specific categories of people are most exposed to crime: young people (16–24 years of age), the unemployed, single parents, people living in rented accommodation and people living in inner-city areas. For the year 1997, the BCS researchers found that there were over 16.5 million offences, but that only a quarter of these had been recorded by the police. That is, they discovered that just half of the crimes of which people stated they had been victims were ever reported, and then only half of these were formally registered by the police (Home Office, 1998a).

Furthermore, criminal activity, crime reporting and the monitoring of crime by the authorities are all extremely skewed (Maguire, 1997). For example, most crime (and therefore most policing) takes place in urban areas. There is an incentive for the victims of property crime to inform the police so that insurance claims can be made. However, this is only worthwhile for those who can afford to take out such insurance in the first place. Crimes of violence occurring in intimate relationships and private situations (especially against women) are extensively underreported.

But, even without the postmodern attack on 'facts', what crime statistics represent may be a deliberately distorted version of the presence of criminal activity and police effectiveness. A number of police authorities in Britain have been accused of cheating in the assessment of how much crime takes place in their area (Davies, 1999). Not only are some offences notified by members of the public to the police not recorded (as has been identified by the BCS), but a number then succumb to 'cuffing'. Cuffing, so-called because the reported infringement 'disappears up the police officer's sleeve', is a tactic used to hide low-level crime such as vehicle damage or petty theft by not logging it in official accounts. This is done by simply ignoring the report, by reclassifying such crimes as theft at work under the non-crime heading of 'lost property', or by lumping together multiple burglaries in a particular street on a housing estate as one event. Allegations against the police have also been made for the way in which they compile clear-up rates. Here the tactic is for an individual arrested for, or convicted of, one crime to be encouraged by the police to take the blame for a series of other (usually similar) crimes, which may not have been carried out by that person. The pay-off for the criminal is the opportunity to attenuate the full force of police evidence in his or her trial, and the pay-off for the police is the 'writing-off' of numerous unsolved crimes.

Although there are notable exceptions of people having disappeared and, if they have been killed, their bodies not having been discovered for a long time – if ever – the police are usually notified of unlawful killings. That is, despite the dubiousness of criminal statistics in general, the official recording of homicides is thought to be largely reliable (Smith & Zahn, 1999). However, as discussed in Chapter 3, this to some extent depends on what is sanctioned as 'murder' in the first place.

Insanity

Mental disorder of one sort or another occurs across the world, and is universally both disabling for sufferers and disturbing for their families and communities, whether this be 'Amok' in Malaysia, 'Pibloktoq' in the Arctic, 'Bena Bena' in New Guinea, 'Imu' in Japan, 'Koro' in China, 'Windigo psychosis' amongst native North Americans or 'schizophrenia' in England. In the USA, some estimates indicate that 28% of the population annually have been classified as experiencing psychological dysfunction (nearly 2% having a serious disorder), whereas others have pointed to a rate of virtually one in two people exhibiting symptoms of a psychiatric disorder at some point in their lives (Cockerham, 1996).

A survey of neurotic psychopathology in Britain, using a sample of 10 000 adults living in private households, found that one in seven adults aged between 16 years and 64 years had a 'neurotic' illness during one specified week (Meltzer et al., 1994). The researchers reported that women were much more likely to suffer from neurosis, but that men suffered from alcohol and drug dependency in far greater numbers. Fatigue, disturbed sleep, irritability and worry were found to be the most common symptoms of mental disorder, anxiety and depression being the most prevalent disorders. Measurements used by the World Health Organisation (WHO), which include not just mortality rates, but also the social cost of premature deaths and morbidity, have indicated that the real burden of psychiatric illness in Western countries accounts for more than that of heart disease and cancer (World Health Organisation, 1999).

Defining 'madness' and its boundaries is, however, not only troublesome, but also quite possibly irresolvable to any degree of certainty or common agreement. Mental disorder overlaps many conceptual borders, but deciding in the first place where these borders lie is also extremely difficult. This has a knock-on effect when attempting to define mental 'health' either as an entity in its own right or as a way of demonstrating (through comparison) what mental 'disease' is:

> The history of madness and mental illness reveals two common (and flawed) definitions of mental health: one that it is the absence of mental illness; the other that it is a state of well-being ... [to] define something by the absence of its opposite is simply a semantic sleight of hand and to define it by substitution is procrastination. Neither option furthers our understanding. (Tudor, 1996, p 21)

Tudor points out that this definitional problematic uncertainty is not helped by the interchangeable usage of the terms 'mental illness' and 'mental health' within professional discourse, or by the perception of these two concepts as being two ends of the same spectrum. Nor are these conceptual dilemmas made any less intractable by the linguistic contortions of political correctness. 'Mental illness' and 'mental disorder' have been displaced by the more acceptable (but infinitely more allusive) expressions 'mental ill-health' and 'mental health problems'.

Historians such as Foucault (1971) and Doerner (1981) have projected the view that, in early modernity, categories of deviance were conflated. This, they argue, resulted in various types of social outcast (for example, vagrants, prostitutes, thieves, murderers and the mad) being incarcerated in the same institution. However, Andrews (1996), using local parish records in London, argues that, from the seventeenth century onwards, a distinction was made between idiocy and insanity, and that in the main the population of institutions reflected this differentiation.

Andrews does acknowledge that there was some degree of confusion, and this is reinforced by Digby's (1996) observation that the law removed idiocy from its definition of lunacy only in the twentieth century. Even in the twentieth century, however, there remained legal ambiguity and imprecision with respect to ailments of the mind. For example, the Mental Health Act 1983 of England and Wales used the rubric 'mental disorder' to cover four categories: (a) mental illness, (b) severe mental impairment, (c) mental impairment, and (d) psychopathic disorder. Explanations for the latter three subdivisions of mental disorder were offered as follows:

> 'severe mental impairment' means a state of arrested or incomplete development of mind which includes significant impairment of intelligence and social functioning and is associated with abnormally aggressive or seriously irresponsible conduct ... 'mental impairment' means a state of arrested or incomplete development of mind (not amounting to severe mental impairment) which includes significant impairment of intelligence and social functioning and is associated with abnormally aggressive or seriously irresponsible conduct ... 'psychopathic disorder' means a persistent disorder or disability of mind (whether or not including significant impairment of intelligence) which results in abnormally aggressive or seriously irresponsible conduct. (Mental Health Act 1983, quoted in Jones, 1985, p12)

Critics of this long-standing legislation have pointed out that not only do key elements of each category (e.g. damaged intellectual and social functioning) appear in all three, but also that these definitions are in fact teleological. That is, disease is explained as behavioural disturbance and vice versa (Jones, 1985). Most significantly, however, mental illness itself was not defined at all, being left to the judgement of clinicians.

It can be argued that mental disorder, and related manifestations of psychological distress, are the foremost health concerns for
Western societies because of the amount of suffering and stigma
involved, the cost of care and incessant human rights violations
(Jenkins et al., 1998). Provocatively, however, the redoubtable psychiatrist Thomas Szasz has gone as far as to oppugn the very existence
of (non-organic) mental disorder and depict the practice of psychiatry as illusionary:

> It is customary to define psychiatry as a medical speciality concerned with
> the study, diagnosis, and treatment of mental illnesses. This is a worthless
> and misleading definition. Mental illness is a myth. Psychiatrists are not
> concerned with mental illnesses and their treatments. In actual practice they
> deal with personal, social, and ethical problems in living. (Szasz, 1972, p269)

Szasz argues that psychiatry has persuaded the scientific
community, the law, the media and the public that the effects of
everyday human difficulties are really diseases (Szasz, 1994). For
Szasz, however, much of what psychiatry deals with is not disease but
'behaviour'. This behaviour is related to problems with living, argues
Szasz, and is not the province of medical science.

The social processes involved in the separation of 'normal'
behaviour from 'abnormal' behaviour are, however, in themselves
inconsistent and transient. For example, homosexuality, alcoholism,
epilepsy and anorexia are all behaviours that have historically
switched backwards and forwards from being embraced within
tolerant notions of normality to being regarded as completely unacceptable. Moreover, a precise rendering of who has legitimacy over
which form of misconduct is equally vaporous. Psychopathic behaviour and sexual abusiveness are two major areas of human misconduct that fall between legal and psychiatric categorisation.

There are even internecine disagreements in the medical profession between, for example, psychiatrists and neurologists. These
stretch back to battles in the mid-nineteenth century over who had
the epistemological right to monopolize care of the mad, and about
madness being the same as, or analogous to, physical illness. Moreover, the neurologists were more in favour of non-asylum care for the
mad than were their psychologically trained colleagues who sought a
power base in institutions. Far from defending the liberty of their

'customers', the neurologists were, however, protecting what they discovered to be an extremely financially rewarding community-based 'business' (Colaizzi, 1989).

There are also notable conflicts in the expectations and practices of other mental health workers. Psychiatric nurses proclaim allegiance to humanistic ideals and advocacy roles, whilst the state and the public demand that they function as institutional caretakers and agents of surveillance in the community. Moreover, tension exists between the criminal justice system, psychiatry and such academic disciplines as sociology with regard to how much 'madness' and 'deviancy' overlap. Furthermore, psychiatrists working in the criminal justice system may disagree with each other about what diagnosis a killer suspected of madness should be given, or may not concur over the presence of insanity at all in cases of homicide (Colaizzi, 1989).

Lawyers and psychiatrists both collude (in the sense that they serve as instruments of control for the state) and compete in terms of which professional group should be sovereign in matters concerning the mentally disordered, both within the mental health service and in the courts. For example, whereas psychiatrists are used as 'expert witnesses' in the judicial process, their opinions – even if united over a diagnosis – may be overridden and purely criminal convictions obtained. In the case of the 'Yorkshire Ripper' in 1981, psychiatrists for both the prosecution and the defence concluded that Peter Sutcliffe's responsibility for his actions was 'diminished' as a result of his paranoid schizophrenia (Busfield, 1996), but the judge put the decision on his mental state to the jury. Sutcliffe was found guilty of murder and rape on a majority verdict, with a recommendation from the judge that he serve a minimum of 30 years in prison. Ironically, a few years into his sentence, Sutcliffe was transferred to a high-security hospital as, apart from being exposed to attacks from his fellow prisoners, his mental condition had deteriorated considerably (Prins, 1995).

The tension that exists between lawyers and psychiatrists is historical, as exemplified by this account from a Professor of Medicine and Mental Diseases at the University of Edinburgh in the 1860s:

> That medico-mental science is often at variance with the doctrines and decisions of the courts and the law is a fact too well known and too generally admitted to need formal proof. (Laycock, 1868, p334)

However, legal-medical relationships surely could not hit a lower note than with the recognition that expert witnesses in the USA are regularly ascribed the pejorative appellation of 'courtroom whores' (Mossam & Kapp 1998). This is presumably because lawyers perceive psychiatrists as being willing to sell the version of their expert opinion that will most satisfactorily meet the interests of the buyer of their services.

The conflation of the categories of mental disorder and criminality are all too apparent in prisons. A significant proportion of the prison population, both awaiting trial and sentenced, are suffering from psychiatric malfunction (Maden et al., 1996; Ramsbotham, 1998). One study, using interviews with prisoners, has indicated that, apart from perhaps an understandable high incidence of neurotic symptoms in prisoners, 14% of women and 10% of men on remand, and 14% of women and 7% of men who had been sentenced, suffered from a psychotic illness such as schizophrenia within the previous year (Office for National Statistics, 1998). Moreover, personality disorder was diagnosed in 31% of remanded and sentenced women, and in 63% of men on remand and 49% of sentenced men.

There is also a much higher rate of suicide in prisons compared with that found in the general population. This is despite a raised awareness of the problem amongst prison staff, the open expression of concern by the Director General of the Prison Service in England and Wales, and the introduction of a number of support schemes (for example, multidisciplinary suicide awareness teams) and access by prisoners to outside support agencies such as the Samaritans (HM Prison Service, 1998). Moreover, the contrast between the non-prison population and those in prison is growing more stark. A 22% rise in self-inflicted death by prisoners was recorded in 1995 in England and Wales, with Scotland heading a European league table of suicides in prisons (Gentleman, 1999).

The occurrence of mental disorder at this level in prisons can be regarded as either a 'psychiatrization of criminality' (an increasing number of prisoners being diagnosed as mentally disordered) or a 'criminalization of psychiatry' (more and more mentally disordered people being classified as criminals). Although the analysis of the rise in mental disorder in prisons may centre on the fight for ideological domination by the various professional groups, Busfield points out that the organisation of health services has had a major effect:

> The reduction of residential provision for the mentally disordered has ensured that some individuals, such as those with alcohol or drug related problems, who might have been treated as disturbed in mind, have instead ended up in prisons within the purview of the criminal justice system. (Busfield, 1996, p56)

The closure of mental hospitals and the scarcity of acute psychiatric beds during the 1990s once again incarcerated those considered to be troublesome because of their disturbed mind together with those confined because of 'wrong-doing'.

Apart from the issues of where madness fits as a category, there is an array of dissimilar perspectives that attempt to discern madness. Explanations of the causes of mental disorder range – as with theories of crime – from the reductionist and positivistic view to social determinism. But identifying causality is not the same as accurate delineation. Although there are classification systems recording a large number of psychological malfunctions, there is no general and agreed operationalization of 'mental disorder' that has application to all circumstances. For example, there are two major classification systems (the American Psychiatric Association's *Diagnostic and Statistical Manual* and the WHO's *International Statistical Classification of Diseases*), both of which regularly revise their contents. This fluidity in the nosology of psychiatric medicine means that what is deemed to be incorporated in the array of mad behaviours in one epoch may not be embraced in ensuing eras. Conversely, what is considered to be either normal or criminal today may be colonized by psychiatry in the future.

Moreover, Szasz illustrates the fallibility of psychiatric nosological systems by exposing the subjective processes that they undergo in their conception. Using the example of the American Psychiatric Association (APA), he observes:

> the various versions of the APA's Diagnostic and Statistical Manual of Mental Disorders are not classifications of mental disorders that 'patients have', but are rosters of officially accredited psychiatric diagnoses. This is why in psychiatry, unlike the rest of medicine, members of 'consensus groups' and 'task forces', appointed by officers of the APA, make and

unmake diagnoses, the membership sometimes voting on whether a controversial diagnosis is or is not a disease. (Szasz, 1994, p36)

Szasz also accuses psychiatry of projecting a fallacious correlation between 'diagnosis' and 'disease'. Diagnoses are fabricated
epithets attributed to 'symptoms' or behaviours, which may or may
not correspond to actual disease entities. For Szasz, there is compatibility in the coupling of the diagnostic designation of 'malaria' with
pathological alterations in the working of the human body, but there
is no such synchronicity between psychiatric diagnostic labels and
the 'illnesses' they purport to represent. This, argues Szasz, is why
some psychiatric ailments (for example, masturbatory insanity)
disappear from the medical textbooks. Mental diseases, states Szasz
(1993), are not literalities but metaphors.

The forced confining in asylums and prisons of the mentally
disordered, both in the past and at present, demonstrates for Szasz
(1998) that although the 'illness' metaphor is used extensively, the
social status of the mad is very different from that of the physically ill.
The mentally disordered, argues Szasz, are treated in this way
because they are assumed to have 'misbehaved' rather than because
they are actually 'sick'.

Mental health policy

Whatever madness is, it not only causes immense personal distress, but
also places society in a predicament over the cost of furnishing treatment and care, the procurement of consistent and credible policies,
and its effect on social stability. Over two millennia, 'reason' has
ascended as the overriding system of belief and has been used to justify
comparatively steadfast social conditions in the developed world:

> Like many other attributes of Western civilisation and intellectual develop-
> ment, modern concepts of mental illness originated with the ancient Greeks
> and Romans. The Greeks, in particular, are noted for formulating a rational
> approach toward understanding the dynamics of nature and society. They
> replaced concepts of the supernatural with a secular orientation that viewed
> natural phenomena as explainable through natural cause-and-effect rela-
> tionships. (Cockerham, 1996, p9)

Since ancient times, the powerful, whether regarded as a unitary
and privileged 'class' or as disconnected groupings dispersed

throughout society, have attempted to maintain social order by exercising control over those deemed to have forfeited their 'reason' (Ingleby, 1982). However, in the fifth century, a mixture of superstitious and religious beliefs filled the ideological chasm left by the fall of the western part of the Roman Empire. The 'middle ages' saw the rise of the Roman Catholic Church and barbarian kingdoms (which were eventually to lead to the formation of nation states in Europe) and was characterized by corruption, warfare, cruelty, epidemics and famine. The consequence for the mentally disturbed of this fusion of Christian and pagan thought in the medieval epoch was the restitution of 'supernatural' explanations, which included both the idea of 'evil' and witchcraft.

However, rationality and reasonableness once again formed the fundamental tenets of those European countries which industrialized, with the eventual spread of reason, science and capitalism to the 'New World'. Mental disorder has come to be viewed as placing in jeopardy the 'health' of 'rational' social systems in a way that no other type of deviancy does. Madness intimidates authority so profusely because unintelligible actions and oratory, particularly if flaunted in the public arena, openly contest social norms based on reason. The exposure to the population of naked 'non-sense' invalidates intellectual deduction and scientific and technological invention. That is, the very credibility and perpetuity of the 'rationalist' paradigm is undermined by the 'crazed' behaviour and thoughts of the insane (Morrall, 1999a). This no more so than when an innocent bystander is inexplicably killed by a psychopath or paranoid schizophrenic.

As Szasz has noted (1998), the response of the powerful to those perceived to be *non compos mentis* has been one of segregation and marginalization. Asylums, built beyond the scrutiny of the 'normal' population, had been in existence since the Middle Ages, but were to grow in number substantially during the nineteenth century (Shorter, 1997). They came to signify material manifestations of exclusionary and Darwinian convictions of the Victorian age. The epoch of 'asylumdom', in which custodial warehouses were used to 'store' sections of the population considered to be 'unreasonable' (Scull, 1993), has been denigrated as an inhuman age:

In 1812, scandal broke when Godfrey Higgins discovered in York Asylum
(of which he was governor) thirteen women in a cell twelve feet by seven feet
ten inches, and that the deaths of 144 patients had been concealed. The
same spring, Edward Wakefield found a side-room in Bethlem hospital
where ten female patients were chained by one arm or leg to the wall. In a
lower gallery (traditionally the area of an asylum where the 'troublesome'
and 'dirty' patients were kept), the pitiable figure of James Norris was found,
confined to the trough where he lay. Norris died of consumption a few days
after his release. (Fennell, 1996, p14)

However, those who initiated asylumdom had not intended to
create the deplorable circumstances experienced in these institutions
by some of their inhabitants. The imposing and forbidding architec-
ture of the insane institution undoubtedly represents an ostentatious
display of the power to expel by the state and psychiatry, but for
many inmates residence in the asylum was a refuge from far worse
conditions at the hands of their relatives. Shorter refers to the 'care'
received by the mad from their families both in Germany and
England in the 1700s:

Before the nineteenth century, looking after the insane was a family affair.
And home care in the world we have lost was a horror story. Anton Muller,
chief of psychiatry at the Royal Julius Hospital in Wurzburg, gave an
account of some of the newly admitted patients. "A youth of sixteen, who for
years had lain in a pigpen in the hut of his father, a shepherd, had so lost the
use of his limbs and his mind that he would lap up the food from his bowl
with his mouth just like an animal". When admitted to the hospital, Muller's
patients ... were routinely found to have "backs beaten blue, with bloody
wounds". One man had been chained by his wife to the wall of their house
for five years, losing the use of his legs ... In England, such patients, if not
chained at home, might be fastened to a stake in a workhouse or poorhouse.
(Shorter, 1997, pp2–3)

A new age of community care arrived in the early part of the
twentieth century in Europe and the USA with the mental hygiene
movement (Goodwin, 1997). This movement encouraged the establishment of various outpatient services. A sharp reduction in the
number of hospital beds, from a peak of 155 000 during the 1950s in
Britain, continued throughout the 1960s and 70s. Community
services were, however, never able to compensate for the loss of many
of the large institutions, and as a consequence, the remaining inpatient services came under intense pressure. For example, admissions

rose from 200 000 in 1983 to 270 100 in 1995 (Sainsbury Centre, 1998). The number of compulsory admissions of patients (under the 1983 Mental Health Act) to National Health Service (NHS) hospitals rose from 15 400 in 1987–88 to 25 100 in 1997–98 (Department of Health, 1998a). During March 1998, 12 700 patients were detained in hospital, of whom 1300 were in high-security psychiatric (special) hospitals. The Mental Health Act Commission, a special health authority with the responsibility constantly to review the operation of mental health legislation, reported that ethnic minority groups were over-represented amongst those psychiatric patients who were detained (Department of Health, 1999a).

A figure of $67 billion was estimated in 1992 to be the cost of treating mental disorder in the USA (Cockerham, 1996). It has been suggested that, in Britain, the financial burden of mental disorder is greater than that of the defence budget, representing 4% of the gross domestic product. The calculation, by health economists at the Institute of Psychiatry in London, of this figure at £32 billion pounds (for the year 1996–97) is based on adding together the figures for wasted productivity (including that lost through suicide), social security payments, the health, local authority and criminal justice services, and informal care (Brindle, 1997).

However, although there is an undeniable difficulty in determining what madness is, and who the mad are, there is less ambiguity about the deranged or 'half-minded' (Thornicroft, 1998) condition of policies for the mentally disordered:

> Services for the mentally ill are in turmoil in many parts of Britain ... with Government plans setting out how mental patients ought to be cared for ... being widely ignored. (Fletcher, 1995)

The mayhem is signified through a never-ending deluge of policy initiatives, legislation and recommendations from reports and inquiries. In the past few decades in Britain, mental health practitioners and managers have been expected to: accommodate the independent sector; disentangle purchasers from providers, and health care from social care; introduce care plans for patients discharged from hospital; offer non-custodial care and treatment to mentally disordered offenders; reduce morbidity and suicide rates; give priority to people placed on supervision registers; implement

new mental health legislation; assess the risk of violence and homicide; provide 'seamless' care or a 'continuum' of care; respond to the
implications of the Patient's Charter; empower users and carers;
audit clinical practice; implement the recommendations of a succes-
sion of reviews concerning the education and roles of psychiatric
nursing; 'assertively outreach' into the homes of patients; and base
medical and nursing practice not on intuition and experience, but on
empirical evidence from randomized controlled trials and experi-
ments.

Moreover, in the late 1990s, a long-term 'modernization
programme' for the NHS began, designed to improve buildings and
equipment, invest in staff training, and procure and develop 'lead-
ing-edge' information technology (Department of Health, 1998b).
Added to this major overhaul of the whole system, and under the
New Labour government's epithet of 'The Third Way', the Department of Health (DoH) launched its objective to renovate all mental
health provision, have a 'root and branch' reassessment of mental
health law and establish guidelines on 'national standards' (Department of Health, 1998c, 1998d, 1998e, 1999b, 1999c). Although
these changes are presented as a way of avoiding the pitfalls of policies based solely on either the asylum or the community, there is in
effect a re-emphasis on institutional care and public safety. That is,
'The Third Way' gives much more weight to acute inpatient hospital
services, secure accommodation and the need to protect both the
public and the mentally disordered by removing 'dangerous' patients
from the community, rather than being a pledge to reinvest in the
policy of care in the community (Warden, 1998a). During the twentieth century, therefore, the mad have been incarcerated, de-incarcer-
ated and, with the advent of post-liberal mental health policies and
legislation, re-incarcerated.

Furthermore, confirming prolonged public anxiety over the
competence of such groups as social workers, general practitioners,
psychiatrists and psychiatric nurses, the mental health disciplines
have been severely criticized for not 'pulling together' (Sainsbury
Centre, 1997). This level of criticism has also been directed towards
the care received by users of psychiatric inpatient services.

In a study of 118 psychiatric units in England and Wales (representing 47% of the total number of inpatient services in NHS trusts),

two major failings were revealed (Ford et al., 1998). First, there was considerable pressure on the acute services (in terms of being able to admit more patients than there were beds), but this was in part created by poor management strategies. Specifically, the study concluded that the policy of sending patients who were compulsorily detained under the Mental Health Act 1983 on short or unspecified leave into the community resulted in these beds being unusable for other patients requiring admission as it was unknown when the 'detained' patients would return. Second, not only was there a serious difficulty in staffing the psychiatric units, which resulted in the overuse of 'bank' or 'agency' nurses, but there was also little interaction with patients in a sizeable minority of the institutions visited:

> On a quarter of the wards there was no nurse in contact with patients at the time of the visit. At the same time, considerable numbers of nurses were engaged in continuous observation, frequent observation, and door duty, but not necessarily in direct contact with patients. (Ford et al., 1998, p1282)

In another survey of care in acute psychiatric wards, information was gathered from over 200 patients about their experiences (Sainsbury Centre, 1998). The conclusions of the investigative team were that although the immediate mental state of the patients improved during their stay in hospital, as measured by the patients' own accounts and objective assessment (using the Brief Psychiatric Rating Scale), they had not had their long-term and individual needs met. The study concluded that hospital care was a 'non-therapeutic intervention' as most of the patients became bored as a result of the absence of structured activity, most had little privacy, and many feared for their personal safety. A recommendation of the study was that acute hospital services should be completely reconstructed.

In research repeating studies of acute mental health services conducted in the 1980s, Higgins et al. (1999) interviewed over a hundred staff and 52 patients, and observed ward activity in 11 sites. These researchers concluded that the education that psychiatric nurses receive does not equip them adequately for working in acute settings. For example, concern was expressed by those interviewed that newly qualified nurses did not have relevant and practical skills for the clinical situations with which they had to deal. Higgins et al. also recorded the fact that the increase in time that senior ward staff spent on paperwork and office duties was 'astonishing'. In 1985, the most senior of these nurses spent a third of their time on this type of work. By 1996, nearly three-quarters of their time was occupied with administrative tasks. Axiomatically, these nurses were in direct contact with patients in 1996 for less than 6% of their working day, compared with nearly 30% in 1986. As a consequence:

> many [patients] had only a passing relationship with nurses who were typi-
> cally in the office writing, telephoning or dealing with unexpected incidents
> in the ward. This resulted in the boredom reported by many patients who,
> when in hospital, felt that they were often left to their own devices. (Higgins
> et al., 1999, p154)

Somewhat confusing, however, are the findings from a 'satisfaction survey' of over 500 users of the psychiatric facilities, including hospital inpatients and those attending outpatient departments, day units and community services (Rogers et al., 1993). Many of the respondents believed that their views were not given adequate attention with regard to the problems they experienced with their treatment in general, and they were ambivalent about the availability and helpfulness of psychiatrists, although nurses were in the main viewed as providing an adequate standard of care. Overall, however, the psychiatric disciplines were 'damned with faint praise'.

Within the context of these wider policy initiatives, the forensic service has its own uncertainties. Indeed, John Gunn, Professor of Forensic Psychiatry at the Institute of Psychiatry in London, has suggested that the service is at a crossroads (Gunn, 1998). Specific concerns in the forensic service are: (a) a significant rise in the number of mentally disordered people contained within prisons (Office for National Statistics, 1998; Ramsbotham, 1998); (b) an increase in the number of suicides by prisoners (Gentleman, 1999); (c) the potential for the human rights abuse of mentally disordered people in the criminal justice system (MIND, 1997); (d) the building of new secure accommodation in the community (Department of Health, 1998f); (e) the privatization of some parts of the service (Beck, 1995; Taranto et al., 1998); and (f) a reorganization of the maximum secure facilities for the mentally disordered following a report on management failure and an 'untherapeutic' environment at Ashworth Special Hospital (Fallon, 1999).

It has also been noted that there are credible innovations in policy and practice within the forensic service. However, there is on the whole a dearth of research and a lack of dissemination of what knowledge has already been accumulated, as well as a general failure of 'communication' both within and across the various institutions that deal with mentally disordered offenders (Ash, 1998; Exworthy, 1998; Gunn, 1998; Mason & Mercer, 1998; Fallon, 1999).

Summary

The conceptual parameters of crime and madness are nebulous and fuzzy, and the organization of care and treatment for the mad is both incoherent and suffering from policy overflow. However, although robust explanations for, and ways of tackling the consequences of, crime and madness have proven intractable, this is no excuse for nihilism. To use an analogy, it may be an intricate and perplexing task to describe an elephant to someone from a culture that has never been in contact with this hardly credible creature, but that should not lead to the conclusion that its existence is dubious. Furthermore, a variability in the cultural and temporal meaning attached to all objects does not diminish the necessity of removing ourselves from the path of a charging bull elephant wherever we are and no matter what the time.

Chapter 2
Disordered offenders

Following the discussion in Chapter 1 about crime and insanity as separate entities, the question of what connects madness to crime is explored in this chapter. The dilemmas surrounding the issue of interpreting 'mad and bad' behaviour are examined, commencing with an account of how the psychiatric and legal professions compete with regard to who has authority over, and responsibility for, those who become known as 'mentally disordered criminals'.

Pivotal episodes and verdicts are presented to illustrate the way in which the criminal justice system and psychiatric medicine have attempted to provide appropriate criteria to judge who is mad and bad. Finally, how the state intends to address the intractable problem of psychopathic behaviour is reviewed.

Contested domains

As has been demonstrated in the example of the trial of Peter Sutcliffe (discussed in Chapter 1), the definitional difficulties with respect to 'criminality' and 'madness' are superimposed onto the combined category of 'mentally disordered offenders'. The overlap between the two categories is, however, not a new phenomenon. In the nineteenth century, Dr Thomson, resident surgeon at the General Prison for Scotland in Perth, observed:

> On the border-land of Lunacy lie the criminal populations. It is a debatable region; and no more vexed problem comes before the Medical Psychologist than this – viz: where badness ends and madness begins in criminals. (Thomson, 1870, p487)

Attempting to define the mentally disordered criminal poses an insuperable quandary involving at one level the courts making decisions about personal responsibility, free will, self-control, maturation, legal liability and punishment and/or treatment. At another level, the frequently contending and internally discrepant beliefs and practices of the law and psychiatry cause further confusion and irresolution. Moreover, the controversy over whether or not the criminal justice system or the psychiatric profession should have province over such disorders as psychopathy continues to produce legislative and political consternation (McCallum, 1997). Indeed, there has been throughout the development of Western civilization, a tension between the law and the medical profession over within whose domain the criminally insane rest.

For Michel Foucault (1988), psychiatry helped to resolve a paradox over the 'intelligibility' of criminal acts from the early part of the nineteenth century onwards. The growing commitment to rationalism and individualism, as a consequence of industrialization, meant that the criminal justice system focused on the personal responsibility of the miscreant. In this setting, a discourse of 'disclosure' is demanded. By the nineteenth century, courts were interested in the criminal as well as in the crime and the penalty. Judges, jurors and lawyers expect to be provided with details not only of the infraction and the immediate circumstances, but also of the personal and social history of the accused. Foucault refers to a case in a French court of a man convicted of kidnapping and killing a child. The man's defence lawyer made a plea against the death penalty, arguing that little about the man had been forthcoming from the interrogations of the police or the court; he asked the question, 'Can one condemn to death a person one does not know?' (Foucault, 1988, p127). The inference here was that only when the crime was made intelligible (through the presentation of 'understandable' aspects of the criminal's biography) could the discipline of the court be justified.

'Unintelligible' crime (in which no motivating factors have been disclosed by the accused or discovered by the court) is to be conceived as not being the responsibility of the perpetrator, and is thereby 'excused' as an act of madness. Recategorized as such, insane murders became the province of psychiatry. Trials of 'monstrous crimes' such as the killing of children for no apparent purpose have allowed psychiatry successfully to penetrate the criminal justice system. Medical experts adjudicating over such crimes have justified the legitimacy of their interventions by demonstrating that no 'reason' could be explicated. Foucault cites two other infamous murders of the nineteenth century:

> In the case of Henriette Cornier, who had decapitated her neighbour's daughter, it was carefully established that she had not been the father's mistress, and that she had not acted out of vengeance. In the case of the woman from Selestat, who had boiled up her daughter's thigh, an important element of the discussion had been, 'Was there or was there not a famine at the time? Was the accused poor or not, starving or not?' (Foucault, 1988, p132)

Presumably, if Henriette Cornier had been known to be sexually consorting with the victim's father, and the cannibal from Selestat had been in a state of abject hunger, the court would have had no hesitation in taking the 'reasonable' course of killing them both.

The history of a legal recognition of insane criminality and thereby reduced culpability, however, dates far further back than the nineteenth century in English law. Andrews et al. (1997) suggest that it has been accepted for as long as anything that could be described as formal English law has existed. They record that, during the rule of King Aethelred in the tenth century, a clear distinction was made between an offence conducted 'of an individual's own free will' and one carried out without him or her 'willing or intending to'.

Daniel Robinson (1996), Professor of Psychology at Georgetown University, traces the history of the mentally disordered offender back even further. Robinson contends that the ancient Greeks and Romans sanctioned an individual's lessened capacity to be held responsible for a crime. In addition, Robinson observes that, throughout the Middle Ages in England and many other parts of Europe, both ecclesiastical and secular courts excused, to a greater or lesser degree, crimes (even murder) committed by the insane. Moreover, according to Robinson, inherent within laws on criminal insanity since ancient times is the acceptance that the law only has jurisdiction over those who are considered to be fully cognisant of their crimes.

Against the background of a general deinstitutionalization of the mentally disordered in the twentieth century, the demarcation of 'bad' from 'mad' has been reified in the specific way in which the criminal justice system works (Colombo, 1997). In Britain, for example, the policy of placing and treating mentally disordered offenders in the community 'whenever possible' became the vogue policy in the early 1990s (Department of Health and Home Office, 1991). Also at this time, a policy was introduced to monitor the mentally disordered going through the courts and steer appropriate cases away from prison into the care of the psychiatric and social services (Home Office, 1990). Some eight years later, more than 100 court assessment and diversion schemes were in operation in England (MIND, 1997). This created a climate in which the incarceration in prison of mentally disordered people was to be a policy of last resort (Peay, 1997).

There is, in effect, an implicit acceptance of 'Penrose's Law' by policy makers. Penrose (1939) argued that the number of people imprisoned rises when the asylum population level falls and vice versa. Decisions of whether or not an offender is sent to a secure hospital or prison have been adjudged to be relatively arbitrary (MacCulloch & Bailey, 1991). Moreover, 'The Terror' of mad murders (see Chapter 8) has affected these reforming and munificent approaches, and the arrival of post-liberal laws and policies has rolled back the programme of community care for all mentally disordered people.

Notwithstanding attempts to decriminalize mentally disordered offenders by using community placements or by helping them to avoid contact with the criminal justice system, the list of mental problems that are dealt with at one time or another by the courts is extensive. It includes not only those categories which are covered by mental health legislation (i.e. neurotic and psychotic illnesses, personality disorder and learning disability), but also drug and alcohol abuse, automatism and sex offending. Furthermore, the courts receive medical advice about the mental state of defendants (psychiatric reports) in mitigation of penalty for a large variety of offences, even though the overall number of cases in which psychiatric reports are requested is only 5% (Prins, 1995).

In Anglo-American criminal justice, 'insanity' has traditionally been used as an admission of guilt but offered as a way of avoiding the usual punishment for a particular crime (Cockerham, 1996). The defendant confesses to the crime but, by reason of insanity, avows that he or she was not responsible for his or her actions. In the main, the defence of insanity only applies either to those who were suffering from a mental disorder at the time of the offence and/or to those who are not competent to stand trial. Where a defendant is found to be unable to understand the charges or help in the preparation of the case by the defence lawyer because of a mental disorder, he or she may be held 'unfit to plead'.

Ironically, the defence of 'insanity' or 'unfit to plead' is adopted prudently as, if accepted, it may result in a far longer spell of incarceration (for example, in a secure hospital) than would have been the case had the conviction been otherwise upheld. In England, however, detention in secure psychiatric accommodation following a successful plea of 'insanity' or 'unfit to plead' is no longer mandatory (except in murder cases) since the implementation of the Criminal Procedure (Insanity and Unfitness to Plead) Act of 1991. The outcome for the offender may thus not be detention (for example, in secure facilities ranging from a psychiatric intensive care unit to a 'special' hospital such as Rampton, Ashworth and Broadmoor): community supervision or guardianship, or even absolute discharge orders, may be enforced.

Having even a severe mental disorder does not preclude an individual from arraignment. If the accused can comprehend the nature of the charges and offer information about the events surrounding the crime, then legally he or she can be dealt with like any other defendant. The fact that an offender has a diagnosed mental disorder does not inevitably mean that this will result in a form of treatment by the court different from that given to the 'normal' offender (Smith & Bailey, 1984). The problem for the courts concerns not merely how to decide whether an accused person is guilty and mad, but whether or not he or she can be absolved because of madness. Interestingly, the British mental health voluntary organization MIND concurs with this dichotomy with regard to criminal responsibility in its campaign to defend the rights of the mentally disordered who may be 'diverted' into high or medium secure psychiatric provision for lengthy periods:

> MIND accepts that it does not necessarily follow that if someone suffers from 'mental disorder' they are therefore not responsible for their actions. There

may be cases where this is so. If people are not responsible for their acts there
must be a system which behaves in a moral and ethical manner towards
them. (MIND, 1997, p2)

Beasts and witches

Contemporary understandings of mental disorder are not transfer-
able absolutely into either the times of the ancient Greeks and
Romans or the Middle Ages. Records of happenings from these
epochs are in limited supply, and in need of careful examination to
verify the stories that are available. However, it would appear that
the diagnosis of insanity was, until quite recently in the history of
Western civilization, based on the notion that the mad were irre-
deemably distinguishable from the rest of humanity. They were a
separate genus from that of 'normal' people, essentially 'wild beasts',
and were as such to be either excluded from the jurisdiction of the
courts (i.e. accessing whatever mental health provision was present)
or dealt with by separate laws and forms of discipline:

> The implicit logic of every system of law [is] that the reach of the law extends
> only to creatures able to comprehend its terms and abide by its prescriptions.
> By this very logic, being human is not enough, for some human beings are so
> lacking in comprehension, so possessed by the ruling power of another, and
> so destitute of personal powers of self-control as to be indistinguishable from
> wild beasts. (Robinson, 1996, p20)

But whereas the dichotomy between 'humans' and 'beasts' had
sprung from ancient Greece, the intolerance and bigotry of the
Christian Church, and the superstitious absurdities of feudal life
generally, were, during the Middle Ages in Europe, to produce a
conflation of categories of behaviour. What we may now consider to
be behaviour that was simply 'inconvenient' or disagreeable, or was
at root madness, had the potential to be reconfigured as sorcery, and
as such could have terrible consequences for the accused.

Marion Gibson (1999) provides the example of the trial of a
young female beggar who was accused of witchcraft in 1612. The
woman, Alizon Device, was accused of making lame a peddler she
had met whilst walking along a road from her home to another
village, and with whom she had a heated argument. Helpfully, the
trial clerk, Thomas Potts, wrote of the trial in much detail. Three

versions, however, appear in his pamphlet: one of the story given by
Alizon Device, a second provided by the peddler, and a third given
by the son of the peddler. We are left unsure of whether or not the
accused had been begging from the peddler or asking to buy his
goods, whether or not he had refused to supply the goods or had
given her the goods, or whether or not the peddler had suffered a
stroke during the altercation, which would account for his lameness.
What we do know, however, is that the peddler's version was
accepted by the courts and that Alizon Device was executed for the
crime of witchcraft.

In such cases as that of Alizon Device, there has to be a sensitive
reading of background considerations such as the social standing of
those involved. That is, being both a woman and a beggar in
medieval times was not likely to lend great weight to one's rendition
of events. Although this did not seem to be so with Alizon Device, it
is probable that many of those determined to be witches were mad,
and much of what was presented to the courts as evidence of sorcery
would at later times be conceived of as signs of insanity. When
women were being charged with witchcraft, this denied them the
opportunity of using insanity as a defence. The content of the accu-
sations of witchcraft were mostly absurd, and torture, used to gain
confessions, excessive. Acts admitted to in these confessions
contributed to the perversity of the ordeal.

The case of Barbara Ruffin in 1611 graphically illustrates the
inhumanity and folly of witchcraft trials. In the German town of
Ellwangen, this 70-year-old woman was arraigned for impiously
verbalizing the Holy Eucharist and using salves to kill cattle and various poisons to murder her own child. Unfortunately for Barbara
Ruffin, not only did her neighbours support the charge, but her
husband also recounted in court occasions in their married life on
which he, when angry, had presumed her to be a witch. She denied
the charges and was subsequently:

> stretched on the rack twice in one day. Still denying her guilt, she was
> tortured again two days later, whereupon she finally admitted not only to the
> desecration of the host but to sexual intercourse with the devil, with whom
> she had entered into a pact. Her spiralling mental anguish and confusion
> only encouraged her tormentors to continue their questioning. (Robinson,
> 1996, p74)

As with Alizon Device, Babara Ruffin was sentenced to death. However, her execution occurred only after five weeks of unremitting interrogation and anguish of the most brutal kind. She was beheaded by the sword.

Offending kings

There have been many celebrated cases in which the courts have tackled the issue of just who is and who is not insane and, if an offender is found to be insane, what should be done with him or her. Throughout the eighteenth century, lawyers and doctors were becoming more aware of the need to define and deal effectively and humanely with the criminally insane. Moreover, public fascination with the issue was never more focused than when the potential or actual victims of insane acts of criminality were British royalty. Ida Macalpine and Richard Hunter, using quotations from historical sources, have examined the attempted regicide of King George III by Margaret Nicholson, a servant from Stockton-on-Tees who believed that the crown was hers:

> On the morning of 2 August 1786 this deluded spinster in her early forties made to stab him [George III] on the pretence of presenting a petition while he was alighting from his carriage at St James's. The weapon was an old dessert knife 'worn very thin', and the blade merely bent against the King's body without inflicting a wound. As she tried to repeat her thrust, a yeoman of the guard caught her and wrested the weapon from her, exclaiming 'She has a knife – is your majesty hurt?' The King 'instantly replied, stroking his hand on his waistcoat – "No, I am not hurt – take care of the woman – do not hurt her, for she is mad."' (Macalpine & Hunter, 1991, p310)

Over a period of week, Nicholson was subjected to interrogations by members of the nobility and political élite, the Prime Minister William Pitt the Younger, the Attorney-General, the Solicitor-General, a father and son team of medical practitioners, three 'elderly matrons' and the Privy Council (which included the Archbishop of Canterbury). The decision was made collectively that she was indeed insane, and, with the King's agreement, she was detained for life in a 'place of safety' (Macalpine & Hunter, 1991). She died in 1828 in Bethlem Hospital at the age of 94, eight years after the death of King George and nearly two decades after he himself had been declared permanently insane.

It was the case of another attempted assassination of the unfortunate George III, this time by James Hadfield, that had a major impact on the way in which madness was dealt with by the courts and eventually brought about an enduring legal test of assessing insanity described as the 'M'Naghten Rules' (discussed below). Hadfield had shot at King George whilst both were attending Drury Lane Theatre on the 15th May of the year 1800, in an apparent attempt to get himself executed for the crime. Unlike Nicholson (or a previous case in which John Frith had thrown a stone at the King's coach), Hadfield was sent to trial. He was accused of treason. He was defended by the best lawyer in England (himself a Scot), Thomas Erskine. It was the line of defence taken by Erskine that was to lay down the cardinal elements of insanity supplications:

> [Erskine] reviewed the range of cases in which the question of insanity had been raised and made the point that a direct 'relation between the disease and the act' must be established to 'deliver a lunatic from responsibility to criminal justice'. (Macalpine & Hunter, 1991, p314)

Erskine stated that Hadfield, although seemingly 'normal' in all other respects, suffered paranoid delusions about the world coming to an end, believed that the continued existence of George III was preventing the coming of the second Messiah, and thought that he must sacrifice himself in order to save humanity. He also believed that his eight-month-old son needed to die in the same cause. Two days prior to his assault on the King, Hadfield had nearly brought about the death of his son by hitting the child against a wall. These delusions, stated Erskine, led to the act for which Hadfield was standing trial and had themselves been the result of previous physical trauma. Whilst fighting for the Duke of York at the Battle of Lincelles in 1783 against the French, Hadfield had sustained an injury that had left permanent damage to his brain, sabre cuts having pierced his skull. During the trial, Erskine drew the attention of the jury to what were described as the 'still visible' cerebral membranes in Hadfield's skull (Robinson, 1996). These injuries, argued Erskine, led to a manifestation of insanity that had a specific focus. That is, Erskine pointed out that the defence of insanity was pertinent where the connection between madness and the transgression was made even if the individual concerned were not completely and permanently insane.

Erskine successfully gained a not guilty verdict on the basis that Hadfield was under the influence of insanity at the time he fired his pistol at the monarch. Thus, the Hadfield judgement meant that the designation of 'wild beast' was now not obligatory for insanity to be used successfully as a defence. Sporadic episodes of madness, or traits of mental dysfunction that left the individual still able to perform competently in all other areas of life, could be claimed in mitigation.

The outcome of the Hadfield case was to propel Parliament into changing the law as the not guilty verdict could have resulted in a 'dangerous madman' being released even if the danger were only spasmodic. Hence, the Safe Custody of Insane Persons Charged with Offences Act of 1800 was passed retrospectively so that Hadfield (and others placed in a new category of offender, the 'criminal lunatics') could be transferred from prison into confinement designated for the insane until 'His Majesty's Pleasure shall be known'.

As with Margaret Nicholson, James Hadfield was sent to Bethlem Hospital. Two years later, Hadfield escaped from Bethlem. Following his near-immediate recapture, he spent 14 years in Newgate Prison before being returned to Bethlem for the remainder of his life. A post mortem confirmed that he indeed had severe damage to his brain as a consequence of his battle injuries (Andrews et al., 1997).

It was usual for the homicidally insane to be incarcerated for life. This could lead to an extraordinary anomaly in the handling of the mentally disordered by the judiciary:

> in Massachusetts in 1879 Charles F Freeman murdered his child under the delusion that the Lord had commanded the sacrifice. The governor sent him directly to the Danvers Lunatic Hospital without trial. By 1883 Freeman had recovered and was brought before the supreme court for a sanity hearing. The alienists gave no conflicting testimony in describing his recovery from the delusion. The result was that he was declared 'not guilty by reason of insanity'. Under the 1873 Massachusetts law, 'when a person is acquitted of murder or manslaughter on the ground of insanity he must, regardless of his condition at the time of his acquittal, be committed to one of the lunatic hospitals for life'. (Colaizzi, 1989, p75)

The illogical containment of the criminally mentally disordered in hospital until death is, however, still (presumably) preferable to a recommendation made by the nineteenth century neurologist William Hammond. Hammond's incomprehensible view was that executing those mentally disordered people who had killed would serve as a warning to other 'lunatics' who might be contemplating homicide (Hammond, 1873). Not only does Hammond's idiosyncratic approach to crime prevention rest incongruously with the causative exegesis of his discipline, but it also appears to be unappreciative of the premise of 'insensibility', which is the basis of 'lunacy'. Throughout the nineteenth century, however, capital punishment was handed out to murderers who were patently mad and diagnosed as such by psychiatric expert witnesses (Colaizzi, 1989).

Delusions and impulses

At various time during the past 200 years, the definition of madness in legal terms, where a homicide has been committed, has centred on a typology produced by French and Anglo-American alienists during the nineteenth century. Perhaps the most influential of these has been Esquirol's (1838) three spheres of disorder, which covers the intellect, emotions and morality, and volition.

Intellectual insanity, characterized by paranoid delusions and command hallucinations, can be seen to be contiguous with what is now categorized as schizophrenia and has been a mainstay of psychiatric diagnosis in cases of murder. Emotional derangement (or 'moral imbecility'), whereby there is an absence of 'conscience' or remorse about killing, and where there may have been gross acts of torture carried out on the victim apparently without motive, has also proved to be an enduring psychiatric diagnosis. Today, the term 'psychopathy' or 'sociopathy' is applied to those who are intellectually intact but without emotional or moral reflection.

The inability to resist a 'homicidal impulse' has been consistently referred to in forensic literature. For example, Dr J Wiglesworth, a British asylum superintendent, wrote in the *Journal of Mental Science* about an event that took place in 1900. It involved two female patients, Hannah Hancox and Mary Grainger, who were (as was practice at the time) employed in his house as domestic servants:

> On the morning in question ... whilst I was at breakfast, I heard some one screaming ... which were loud and persistent ... I hastily ran upstairs to see

what was the matter. On arriving at the top (my house is a high one of three
stories) I found the woman Hancox lying on her left side on the stone land-
ing at the top of the stairs, and Grainger (the other woman) kneeling over
her cutting at the neck with a knife. This bald statement of fact conveys but
little idea of the horrible nature of the scene. (Wiglesworth, 1901, p336)

Wiglesworth goes on to describe the savagery of the attack by
Grainger, which produced wounds leading to the death of Hancox.
He believed that, but for his intervention, Grainger would have
succeeded in cutting off Hancox's head. On examination after the
event, Wiglesworth found Grainger to be, although somewhat
agitated, coherent and rational, without remorse and in full knowledge of what she had done (as she had planned the killing). That
morning, however, and on at least one previous occasion, she had
experienced an uncontrollable urge to kill somebody. Following a
court appearance, Grainger was transferred to Broadmoor Asylum.

Murderous implulses were initially considered to represent a
separate disorder. However, although occasionally rejuvenated as a
discrete homicidal phenomenon, this became identified as a symp-
tom of psychiatric disorder, principally schizophrenia (although it
has also be allied with psychopathy). Other volitional disturbances,
thought to indicate dangerousness, have at various times been attributed to obsessional-compulsive neurosis and the 'mania' part of
manic depressive psychosis.

Epilepsy has also been implicated in volitional homicide. Dr
Smith, physician for mental disorders at the Charing Cross Hospital in
London, reported in 1901 what he considered to be a case of 'epileptic
homicide'. This involved Charles Canham, who had a history of 'fits'
that had commenced during his army service in Africa during the late
1800s. He was to remember nothing of the killing of his wife and child:

On November 29th, 1900, prisoner [Canham] and his wife went to bed at
11pm, the child sleeping in the same room. At 7.30 the next morning the
eldest daughter went as usual to call her father and mother and to take them
cocoa. She knocked, but received no answer ... eventually assistance was
obtained, and at 12.30 the door was broken open. The wife was then found
to be dead in bed with four penetrating wounds in the scull, as well as three
other contused wounds ... the child was found to have its throat cut so extensively that all the vessels and the trachea were completely divided, while the
wound had extended through an intervertebral disc, and had even gone into
the spinal cord. (Smith, 1901, pp528–9)

Dadd and M'Naghten

During the nineteenth century in England, dangerous and criminal patients were contained within the ordinary county and borough asylum. Bethlem had a specialist 'department', which in 1852 housed over 100 inmates, this at the time representing nearly a quarter of England's incarcerated criminally insane population (Andrews et al., 1997). The first purpose-built asylum for the criminally insane (Broadmoor) was opened for women in 1863 and for men a year later. Broadmoor, built by the military engineer Sir Joshua Jebb, was similar in architectural style to a prison. Amongst the inmates transferred from Bethlem to Broadmoor (where he eventually died in 1886) was the artist Richard Dadd, who in 1843 was to be 'sensationalized' in the newspapers for the 'insane killing of his father'.

Dadd had joined the Royal Academy Schools in London at the age of 20 and was to gain the reputation of an accomplished draughtsman and painter. Some five years later, whilst touring in Egypt with his work, he began to suffer increasingly from depression and psychotic symptoms:

> On his return [to England], his actions became unpredictable and occasionally violent. He was now watchful and suspicious, obsessed with Egyptian mythology. Increasingly he believed that he was being persecuted by the devil's minions and that voices were influencing him in his own mission to rid the world of the devil. His landlady became afraid of his bizarre behaviour, although Dadd's father persistently claimed that there was nothing wrong with his son despite the advice of Alexander Sutherland, physician at St Luke's, who advised that Dadd should be restrained. Shortly after Sutherland had been consulted, Dadd called his father and suggested a walk in the country near Cobbam to help him clear his mind. On the walk Dadd repeatedly stabbed his father with a spring knife he had brought along for the purpose, convinced that his father was the devil. (Andrews et al., 1997, pp504–5).

Daniel M'Naghten's case, in the same year as Dadd's, was to have the greatest impact on the law relating to insanity. M'Naghten, a carpenter from Glasgow, suffered paranoid delusions directed toward members of the Tory political party. He was charged in 1843 with the homicide of Edward Drummond (who took five days to die) whom he had shot by mistake. His intention was to kill the Tory Prime Minister Sir Robert Peel (1788–1850), to whom Drummond was the private secretary. After the presentation of medical evidence, the trial judge indicated to the jury that he believed the case for the defence to have been established so as to leave no doubt as to M'Naghten's madness. M'Naghten was found 'not guilty on the ground of insanity' and also became an inmate of Bethlem.

After the M'Naghten trial, however, there were some influential dissenters from the verdict. Queen Victoria, who had herself been the target of a number of assaults, was to complain in a letter to Sir Robert Peel that she (and most of her subjects) believed M'Naghten to be conscious of what he had done and therefore not insane (Robinson, 1996, p164).

Subsequent to the M'Naghten trial, to succeed in a claim of insanity, aside from a starting point of assuming that all humans are sane unless proven otherwise, there are three points to be substantiated (Cross et al., 1988). First, the accused must have been suffering from a 'disease of the mind' (whether the aetiology of such a disease was organic or functional, and whether transient, enduring, susceptible to treatment or incurable) at the time of the unlawful deed. What is excluded as a satisfactory 'disease of the mind' for the purpose of the M'Naghten Rules are those mental disturbances which come about as the consequence of external factors such as violence, drugs, alcohol, hypnosis and hypoglycaemia. Second, the disease of the mind must produce a 'defect of reason' beyond simple moments of absentmindedness or confusion. Third, this reasoning deficiency means that the offender either did not know the nature and quality of his or her actions or, if knowing this, was unaware of the wrongfulness (in the 'moral' rather than merely 'legal' sense) of these actions.

There has, however, never been universal acceptance of the M'Naghten rules. For example, some 20 years after M'Naghten, in his vitriolic side-swipe at the way in which the courts undervalued medical opinion, and at the (English) judges who produced the M'Naghten Rules, Laycock highlights the discord between and amongst the medical and legal professions about the saliency of insanity as absolution for murder:

> the present state of our jurisprudence in regard to persons mentally incapable and irresponsible is in every way defective ... [The] doctrines laid down in 1843, by the twelve English judges, are of this obsolete character. (Laycock, 1868, pp344–5)

The importance of the M'Naghten Rules has declined with subsequent legislation. Medical jurisprudence has gradually, and not without a great deal of controversy and ambiguity, grown in significance. Expert medical opinion was to displace attempts to obtain universal rules governing mental disorder in criminal law.

Moreover, 'diminshed responsibility' can now be used in mitigation against a murder conviction. If found culpable but suffering from diminished responsibility, the lesser charge of manslaughter may be instituted. This was introduced into English criminal law in the 1957 Homicide Act:

> Where a person kills or is party to the killing of another, he shall not be convicted of murder if he was suffering from such abnormalities of mind (whether arising from a condition of arrested or retarded development of mind or any inherent causes or induced by diseases or injury) as substantially impaired his mental responsibility for his acts and omissions in doing so or being a party to the killing ... A person who but for this section would be liable, whether as principal or as accessory, to be convicted of murder shall be liable instead to be convicted of manslaughter. (The Homicide Act 1957, section 2, quoted in Smith and Hogan, 1988, p203)

There have also been other interesting modifications to the M'Naghten test. In Virginia in the USA, for example, the addition of the notion of 'irresistible impulse' to the M'Naghten criteria provided emotional elements to an otherwise mainly 'intellectual' judgement about the person's state of mind (Cockerham, 1996). In 1994, Lorena Bobbitt became famous for cutting off her husband's penis. She gained an acquittal on the basis of 'temporary insanity'. Her defence was that years of alleged physical and emotional abuse, and spouse rape, had led her to succumb to an 'irresistible impulse'. Benefiting from advances in corrective surgery, which enabled his penis to be reattached, the husband, John Wayne Bobbitt, was to succumb to his own 'irresistible impulse' by featuring in pornographic films.

Psychopaths

The law and psychiatry clash over definition and classification most obviously and publicly when it comes to the 'psychopath'. Terms such as 'psychopathy', 'personality disorder' and 'sociopathy' are often used interchangeably. In English legal documents (for example, the 1983 Mental Health Act), 'psychopathy' is adopted, whereas the WHO and the APA favour their own variations of the designation 'personality disorder'. However, the term 'sociopath', with its greater emphasis on the detrimental effects of society (rather inherent psychological disturbances) than on the behaviour of individuals, is also in general use, particularly in the USA.

What constitutes psychopathy is not clear as it is an all-embracing category covering many different types of antisocial behaviour and can be described as the deviancy classification of last resort even within the residual category of madness. Disordered personality traits include: paranoid and schizoid symptoms; antisocial, histrionic, impulsive and inadequate behaviour; emotional instability, impulsiveness, dependency and shallowness; and passivity (Marlowe & Sugarman, 1997).

Moreover, there may also be the contamination of dual or multiple diagnosis, whereby an individual can be said to have a personality disorder and one or more other mental illnesses. Alternatively, manifestations of underlying personality disorder (such as uncontrollable aggression, alcoholism, drug abuse and addictive gambling) may be what brings the sufferer to the attention of either the psychiatric services or the courts.

The debate about what can be deemed to be a personality disorder reflects the general difficulty encountered in arriving at any consensus on the nature of all mental abnormalities. Apart from the complication of trying to delimit 'normal' personality, there is, however, a particular dilemma with this type of disorder because sections of the profession of psychiatric medicine openly declare their lack of commitment to this area of work. The reasons for such a reluctance to deal with psychopathic disorder are indicated by Marlowe & Sugarman:

> They [people with personality disorder] can be difficult to treat, complicate the management and adversely affect the outcome of other conditions, and exert a disproportionate effect on the workload of staff dealing with them.
> (Marlowe & Sugarman, 1997, p176)

Moreover, there has been dispute not only over how to treat disorders of the personality, but also over whether some or all forms are even susceptible to treatment (Warden, 1998b). In England, neither the 1983 Mental Health Act nor the 1995 Mental Health (Patients in the Community) Act insists that the psychiatric disciplines have to accept responsibility for those afflicted by a disorder of their personality if they are considered to be 'untreatable'. The case of Michael Stone (referred to in Chapter 8), diagnosed as suffering from a personality disorder, illustrates the point well. Stone was given three life sentences for the murder of Linda Russell and her six-year-old daughter Megan Russell, and for the attempted murder of her other daughter, Josie Russell. Stone had a long history of violent tendencies and had previously been dealt with by the mental health services. He was allegedly refused his own request for admission to a psychiatric hospital only days before the crime (Duce & Frean, 1998).

The Stone case was somewhat complicated by revelations that one of the key witnesses admitted telling 'a pack of lies' in his evidence against Stone, and that there were discrepancies in his diagnosis. This led to an appeal and police investigation, as well as an independent review of the case by the DoH focusing on the actions of the mental health practitioners involved.

Whatever further insights are gained into this case, the effect of it on mental health legislation and policy, and criminal law, has been to encourage the psychiatric disciplines and/or the criminal justice system to embrace a far more proactive stance in dealing with the psychopath. Moreover, this and other similar harrowing incidents pushed the British government into accepting that there are thousands of people living in the community who are a risk to the public, or will be so on release from prisons and psychiatric institutions. This statement from the British Home Secretary Jack Straw testifies to the existence of this danger, as well as to the failures of both the mental health services and the legal system to resolve their differences over in whose domain the psychopath belongs:

> There is a group of dangerous and severely personality disordered individuals from whom the public are not properly protected, and who are neither restrained effectively by criminal law nor mental health provisions. (Straw, 1999, p1)

To curb the freedom of this group – made up of a mixture of child abusers, rapists, the excessively violent and murderers – a number of proposals have been made by the British government. Principally, key figures in the area in which the offender lives or is to live on discharge (for example, police officers, probation officers, head teachers, health and social service workers, and representatives of the local community) are to be notified of the whereabouts of the dangerous person and of the plans the authorities have for him or her. To follow are to be changes in the law to detain members of this group indefinitely in either prison, secure psychiatric units and hospitals, or specially built accommodation (Home Office, 1999). Those who will not be covered by these new laws may be housed within these institutions on a voluntary basis. Some who have not committed any offence may be arrested and confined.

Summary

Despite hundreds of years of debate on who the criminally insane are and what should be done about them, equivocation persists (Webb & Harris, 1999). Public and governmental disquiet about dangerous people living in the community demonstrates that, at the end of the twentieth century, neither psychiatry nor the law had adequately resolved the issue of disordered killers, nor even that of in whose professional sphere they should be embraced. Mental health and criminal justice legislation and policies in the third millennium will continue to grapple with this contentious area of human conduct.

Chapter 3
Killing people

In the previous two chapters, some of the difficulties in achieving concrete understandings of crime and mental disorder have been highlighted. What then can be said about homicide? Are there similar obstacles to the accurate delineation of 'killing'?

This chapter begins with a discussion of when killing is acceptable and when it is not, and of the significance of official statistics on homicide. An overview of known characteristics of homicide is then presented – who it is that does the killing; the reasons for such a high clear-up rate by the police in cases of murder; and where you are likely to be killed. Certain types of murder, for example the killing of children, multiple and serial killings, and the anomaly of infanticide, are then examined. The phenomenon of 'state homicide' is also addressed. In the last section, data referring to the number of mentally disordered people who kill are examined in depth.

Legal and illegal killing

As with most types of criminal and deviant behaviour, ascertaining accurate definitions and agreed data with respect to murder has proven troublesome. Thomas Szasz's view is that law makers do not uncover but 'invent crimes' (Szasz, 1993). From this viewpoint, killing in itself may not be considered to be a crime, but only those forms of murder that are unsanctioned by the state and its regulatory bodies. For example, the mass extermination of civilians is, depending on its legal status, either 'genocide' or, when authorized by governments and therefore legitimized, a 'military necessity'. Moreover, in time of warfare, the conqueror has the power of veto over which events can be classified licit and which can be vilified. During the Second World War, the Nazi 'blitz' of London was compared unfavourably with the Royal Air Force blanket bombing of Dresden in terms of its moral standing by the victorious allies.

In 1999, Serbian political and military leaders were indicted by the International Court of Justice at the Hague, set up by the Security Council of the United Nations. The then Prosecutor of the Court, Louise Arbour, announced that the Serbian leaders (including the President of the Federal Republic of Yugoslavia, Slobodan Milosevic) were to be charged with 'crimes against humanity' and 'violations of the laws and customs of war' as decreed by the Geneva Conventions. These crimes and violations consisted of the deportation (i.e. 'ethnic cleansing') of a large number of the population of Kosovo-Albanians and the murder of thousands of men, women and children whose bodies have been found in mass graves throughout Kosovo. The Serbian leaders were held to have been ultimately responsible for the regular troops, paramilitary forces, and 'police officers' who carried out these atrocities.

But how do these crimes by the Serbs compare with the calculation of 'collateral damage' (i.e. the killing of non-combatants) prior to military action taken by the leaders of NATO, against whom the Serbian forces were engaged? Operation 'Allied Force' started on the 24th March 1999. More than 900 NATO aeroplanes dropped at least 25 000 bombs over a 78-day period. According to NATO's own figures, 1400 Serbian civilians, as well as 5000 members of the Serbian armed forces, were killed (Norton-Taylor, 1999). Killed also were scores of Albanian Serbs by NATO's 'friendly fire'. Can the murder of non-military personnel on one side of a war be defended morally as an inescapable consequence of 'humanitarian' goals whilst the killing carried out by the other side is decried as the unpardonable act of a despicable tyrant?

The meaning given to the deed of killing in times of war will alter depending on the motive, but how that motive is regarded (i.e. as either honourable or amoral) will be influenced by such variables as the status and power of the perpetrator. It will also rely on the manner in which accounts of the killing are disseminated to the home and world audience. All sides in modern warfare appreciate the need to utilize the services of media 'spin doctors'. These are used to present an interpretation of events that, as far as possible, ensures a sympathetic response from the public in whose name the killing is being conducted, and to reduce the possibility of the enemy gaining assistance (militarily or morally) from other countries by not appearing to be the aggressor.

The legal category of homicide in English law includes the offences of murder, infanticide and manslaughter. Taking the classic definition of murder used in English law, reference is made to the unlawful killing with malice aforethought of 'any reasonable creature *in rerum natura*' (i.e. a living human being). 'Manslaughter' refers to unlawful killing when it is judged that there was an absence of the intention to kill, or substantial mitigating circumstances such as severe provocation or an 'abnormality of mind'. When the latter is applicable, a verdict of manslaughter due to 'diminished responsibility' may be given.

There are patently enormous problems in assessing whether or not the indicted individual intended to kill, whether he or she was induced to kill by the actions of the victim, or whether or not he or she can be held accountable for the killing. There are also fundamental issues concerning when the victim actually dies and what can reasonably be thought to be 'human life'. There was in English law an arbitrary limit of one year and one day on when the victim could be considered to have died from the (intentional) actions of the perpetrator. That is, prior to the Law Reform (Year and a Day Rule) Act of 1996, a killer was not found guilty of murder if the victim lived – or was kept alive artificially – beyond this period, even if the accused set out deliberately to take that person's life.

However, deciding just who can and who cannot be considered to be a 'reasonable creature' produces a dilemma that demands a subjective assessment of the beginning and cessation of human life. That is, the perimeters of human existence are not steadfast, and hence verification of the extinguishing of a person's life may not be categorical:

> The only problems are at what stage in the process of birth a foetus becomes a person; and at what stage in the process of death a person becomes a corpse. It is not murder to kill a child in the womb or in the process of leaving the womb ... The tests of independent existence which the courts have accepted are that the child should have an independent circulation, and that it should have breathed after birth. But there are great difficulties with these

tests ... Similar problems could arise as to the moment at which life ends. Is P
dead, and therefore incapable of being murdered, if his heart has stopped
beating but a surgeon confidently expects to start it again ... Is P dead if he is
in a 'hopeless' condition and 'kept alive' only by an apparatus of some kind?
(Smith & Hogan, 1988, pp310–11)

With the advance of modern medical science, there is further
blurring of 'life' and 'death'. Not only are there far more sophisticated technologies for detecting signs of cardiovascular and cerebral
activity in an otherwise 'dead' person, and methods for bringing the
dead back to life, but also the artificial elongation of life can be for
perpetuity.

As mentioned in Chapter 1, homicide statistics, compared with
other criminal data, are considered to be accurate and complete, but
there is a strong argument for the disaggregation of the homicide
statistics, as making any judgement on the overall figures is meaning-
less given the complex socio-economic and cultural make-up of both
the killers and victims (Hawkins, 1999).

Moreover, there are three sets of data with respect to homicide.
One set refers to the number of deaths considered at the time of
discovery by the police to be the result of unlawful killing. Another
set are those which are recorded as homicide within the active judicial
process of prosecution. Finally, there is the actual sum of convictions.
Hence, it is not possible to be certain of how many people have at
any one point been murdered as some deaths perceived to be the
result of homicide can be later reclassified as, for example, acciden-
tal. These sets of figures, however, tend to follow a parallel trajectory.
Furthermore, none of the data reflect when the crime took place as
some convictions may be related to murders committed years previously. Moreover, the number of offences of homicide recorded by the
police does not correspond to the number of people arrested for this
crime as not only are there situations in which no-one is appre-
hended, but also more than one person can be charged with a particular murder. Nor do the statistics take account of miscarriages of
justice that might be uncovered at a later date.

Incredibly, society tolerates homicide, and accepts the purpose-
ful killing of innocents, as inevitable. Most murders are committed
by someone known to - or possibly even loved by – the victim. Tens
of thousands of deaths per annum throughout the world are vindi-
cated as being 'understandable' in the circumstances, perhaps the

consequence of financial enticement, hormonal imbalance or unbridled possessiveness:

> An amateur jockey was stabbed to death by her jealous lover as she collected
> her belongings from the home they shared ... Michael Parker could not
> accept that his four-year affair with Fiona Barnes, 28, a vet's daughter who
> ran a livery stable, was over. He stabbed her repeatedly in the heart with a
> steak knife. (Jenkins, 1998)

Of course, under certain conditions, society actually promulgates the slaying of large numbers of people. During periods of warfare, a hero status is awarded to the most successful of socially sanctioned assassins. In some countries, a covert or overt policy of mass execution has been adopted by governments in order to address particular forms of criminal activity (drug dealers in China), racial impurity (the eugenic practices of Nazi Germany, intertribal massacres in Rwanda, and 'social reconstruction' in Stalinist Russia and Pol Pot's Cambodia) and civil unrest (colonial India under British rule, and Sadam Hussain's butchery of Kurds in Iraq).

In the social system that upheld apartheid in South Africa, the political party in power and the security services were imputed to have worked together in order to 'neutralize' a large number of fellow citizens who were opponents of that system (Whitaker, 1998). Following the collapse of apartheid, however, the relationships of alleged allies, now under the gaze of a new political élite with different mores, turned sour:

> Eugene de Kock, the death squad leader dubbed Prime Evil by his
> colleagues, yesterday came face-to-face with P W Botha, his master and
> former President ... De Kock, 49, who is serving 212 years for a double
> murder and fraud ... the man who took scores, perhaps hundreds of lives
> during more than 20 years in the police force and in battles with 'terrorists'
> in Namibia, launched into a tirade of contempt for the National Party,
> headed for much of his career by Mr Botha. (Kiley, 1998)

However, the post-apartheid government of Nelson Mandela also had to face uncomfortable publicity about its own history. The 'Truth and Reconciliation Commission' was set up in an attempt to assuage any outbursts of vengeance by the new regime against their former opponents, as well as to generate forgiveness on all sides, through the process of confession without the risk of prosecution. It examined the conduct of the African National Congress (which fought against apartheid both politically and militarily) during the period 1960-90 and described 'gross human rights violations', including torture and murder, by its members (Smith & Beresford, 1998).

Moreover, political expediency can dramatically alter the expected life course of those convicted of the most horrendous of crimes:

> Two IRA killers, jailed for the gruesome murder of two British soldiers 10 years ago, were yesterday free under the Good Friday Agreement ... [The killers] played key roles in the abduction and beating of corporals David Howes and Derek Wood after they drove into an IRA funeral cortege in Andersontown, west Belfast, in March 1988. They were jailed for murder, with a recommendation that they serve a minimum 25 years ... The releases bring to 215 the number of convicted terrorists freed under the agreement. (Mullin, 1998)

There is, therefore, much enigma over what is a legitimate and what is an illegitimate killing.

Certainties about murder

What we can be sure of is that most homicides are committed by men and that over two-thirds of those murdered are also men. The victim is frequently known to the killer. Half of all male victims and three-quarters of female victims have known their killers. Nearly half the women victims are killed by a present or former intimate partner. However, there has been a decline in married partners who kill compared with unmarried lovers.

The police arrest and conviction rate for murder, compared with that of other crimes, is, at approximately 90%, very impressive. This is due primarily to the closeness of the victim to his or her killer. That is, it is to the previous and current lovers that the police first turn in their investigations. It is also a consequence of murders carried out by lovers being, although possibly premeditated, conducted in a state of emotional turmoil and therefore not necessarily being well planned. In such circumstances, motives are far more likely to be ascertained (the victim perhaps having had a sexual affair with another person or having threatened to terminate the relationship), and clues are more likely to be left at the scene of the crime.

Moreover, developments in forensic science now allow for fragments of evidence that would otherwise not be of any use to the prosecution to be used to establish connections between the killer and evidence from the scene of the crime. DNA testing permits microscopic traces of human discharge and skin debris left at the scene of the crime to be analysed. This means that unsolved cases of murder that have been 'closed' for many years can once again be examined, using the evidence collected at the time to compare with the DNA of old or new suspects.

With respect to where killings take place, one is far less likely to be murdered in the European cities of Brussels, Athens, Rome, Dublin and London than in the US cities of Washington DC, Philadelphia, Dallas, Los Angeles and New York, the South Africa city of Johannesburg or the Russian Federation capital of Moscow. In the USA in 1993, there were 24 456 murders and over one million aggravated assaults, the most common form of serious violent crime, which includes rape (Riedel, 1999).

Zahn & McCall (1999) have assessed the trends and patterns of homicide in the USA from 1900 to 1996. They conclude that the 1980s and 90s had the highest rate of homicide, and the 1950s the lowest. The vast majority of violent crimes (including homicide and rape) in the USA are intraracial, mostly black Americans assaulting and killing other black Americans (Clinard & Meier, 1995). The minority of murders not committed by black Americans against other black Americans are perpetrated by whites against whites.

In addition, it is people within the lower stratum of the social hierarchy who carry out most of the violent crime and homicide in the USA, Australia and Britain. As most murders are committed by those known to the victim, it follows that most victims are from the same lower social group in these countries (Levi, 1997). Moreover, evidence from the USA indicates that there are distinctions to be made between lower-working-class murderers and middle-class murderers. The further the murderer is up the social hierarchy, the more likely he or she is to have deliberated for some considerable time over his or her crime, and to have a motive of personal gain (Clinard & Meier, 1995).

The USA is, however, nowhere near the top of the international table of homicide rates (LaFree, 1999). Colombia is the country with the highest homicide rate in the world (89.5 per 100 000 of the population in 1991), nearly four times that of Puerto Rico (22.5 per 100 000 of the population in 1991), the next highest. Mexico, the Russian Federation, Kazakstan, Latvia, Estonia and Belarus all have higher rates than the USA. England and Wales, Ireland and Japan have very low rates (0.6 per 100 000 of the population in 1991), Malta being at the bottom of the table (0.3 per 100 000 of the population in 1991).

In England and Wales during 1997, there were 738 deaths recorded initially as homicide (Home Office, 1998b). This represents a very steep increase from a figure of 315 per year in the 1950s and 337 in the 1960s (mean averages). Children under one year of age are the age group most at risk of being killed. The most regularly used methods of killing are sharp instruments, strangulation, and hitting or kicking. Only a minority of victims (usually under 10%) are slain by bullets.

The number of murders globally, and its burden on global public health, is immense and growing. For example, there was in 1990 an estimated figure of over half a million murders world wide, but this is expected to rise to one million by the year 2020 (Mercy & Hammond, 1999). Amongst the 15–44-year age group, murder is the third leading cause of death.

These are, however, officially defined and recorded statistics. In times of civil strife, such as the break-up of Yugoslavia and the consequential wars involving Bosnia-Hertzegovina, Croatia, Serbia and Kosovo, the number of innocent civilians killed by soldiers, 'police officers' and insurgents (representing the various warring factions), or by other civilians, can only be vaguely estimated.

There is, of course, no chance of reoffending if a convicted murderer has received a death sentence (and it has been carried out). However, only a very small number of convicted murderers reoffend following their release from prison. The number of 'repeat killers' out of all of those who have murdered and are living in the community is estimated to be 0.03% (Levi, 1997). That is, killing does not become a 'career', although up to 20% of discharged murderers do go on to commit other crimes. This may simply reflect judicious sentencing and discharge procedures in that potential repeat killers remain in custody.

Special murders

Certain murders are *sui generis* because of who the victim or the killer is, or as a consequence of the particular characteristics of the crime. For example, aberrant types of murder include the killing of children, children killed by children, and multiple killings by people without the political motives associated with genocide. Moreover, in both the public conscience and the judicial process, certain killers are regarded as 'special' because they are viewed as exceptionally and permanently dangerous.

Ania Wilczynski (1997), in her account of the killing of children of all ages by their parents or parental surrogates (filicide), suggests that there is an underestimation of these types of murder and that the figure may be as high as five times that recorded in official statistics. Moreover, although extremely controversial, one research study in Britain conducted by a leading paediatrician has indicated that a small percentage of children diagnosed as having suffered from 'cot death' may in fact have been murdered – usually by their mothers (Meadow, 1999). According to Professor Sir Roy Meadow, coroners and pathologists are under too great a pressure to ascertain the cause of death in order to reduce psychological stress on the families of the dead child. In addition, he suggests that medical and nursing staff are not sensitive to signs of impending abuse (and potential homicide) when faced with harassed young mothers who attend paediatric units for no apparent genuine reason.

The killing of a young child may, on the face of it, both be the most heinous of crimes and justify a much greater punishment than any other type of murder. This would seem to be particularly warranted where the killer is a parent of the victim. In English Law, however, there is a special category (i.e. infanticide) for the killing of an offspring by the mother. A woman will not be held fully responsible for her actions if, at the time of the crime, medical evidence suggests that she was mentally unstable because of the psychosomatic aftermath of giving birth to any of her children:

Section 1 of the Infanticide Act 1938 provides that where a woman by any wilful act of omission causes the death of her child, being a child under 12 months, in circumstances which prima facie amount to murder, but at the same time of such an act or omission the balance of her mind was disturbed by reason of her not having fully recovered from the effects of giving birth to the child, or by reason of the effect of lactation consequent upon the birth of the child, she is guilty of infanticide, an offence punishable in the same ways as manslaughter. By Section 1(2) of the Act, where a woman is tried for the murder of the child under the age of 12 months, it is open to the jury to return a verdict of not guilty of murder but guilty of infanticide. (Cross et al., 1988, p261)

A mother can, therefore, either be charged with infanticide, or the offence of killing a child whilst psychologically unbalanced can be used as a defence against the accusation of murder. Unlike the defences of insanity and diminished responsibility, however, the evidence of a 'disturbed mind' presented by the defence has to be disproved by the Crown. Moreover, the infanticide legislation can be viewed as providing further advantage to the defendant as there needs to be a lower level of mental disorder established than for diminished responsibility. Wilczynski (1997) regards this level of leniency as being without precedent in criminal law. If found guilty of infanticide, women are generally given probation with a requirement to receive medical treatment.

The phenomenon of the 'child killer of children' hit the headlines in 1960s Britain with the deaths of three-year-old Brian Howe and four-year-old Martin Brown. Mary Bell, herself only 11 years old, was convicted of the manslaughter of these two children and sentenced to life imprisonment. She was released in 1980 with a new identity, but in 1998 she was to gain large-scale media attention by cooperating with the author Gitta Sereny in the publication of her life story. The phenomenon of the child-killer was again to appal as well as fascinate the public in the 1990s with the murder of James Bulger by two 10-year-olds. In 2000, six-year-old Kayla Rolland was shot dead by a same-age classmate in the USA. However, far from being a rare event, Herschel Prins (1995) makes the point that even infants, if frustrated, indulge in 'murderous rage'. Moreover, once again the official statistics cannot be wholly trusted as the law on the age of criminal responsibility does not register as homicide those deaths which are caused by the deliberate actions of children if they are under a certain age.

Multiple-victim killings have presumably occurred since the beginning of human group life. The killing of numerous people by a lone assassin on one occasion, or over a period of time, became recognized as a world-wide phenomenon in the 1980s. For the most part, these killings have involved firearms. A growing number are being carried out by children on children. In 1997, more than 6000 American children were expelled for carrying guns or explosives on the premises of their school (Marshall, 1998).

Single incidents of mass murder have included: in 1987, the killing of 16 people in the English village of Hungerford; in 1989, the killing of 14 young women at the University of Montreal; in 1990, the killing of 11 people (including children) at the New Zealand seaside hamlet of Aramoana; in 1996, the killing of 16 children who were attending school in the small Scottish town of Dunblane; in 1996, the killing of 35 people in the Australian tourist resort of Port Arthur, Tasmania; in 1997, the killing of six people and the injuring of five others at the New Zealand ski resort of Raurimu; in 1998, the killing by a 15-year-old boy of his parents and two other teenagers, as well as the wounding of nearly two dozen other schoolchildren, in Springfield, Oregon; in 1999, the killing of 12 schoolchildren and a teacher in the Denver suburb of Littleton, Colorado by two of their classmates (who also died); in 1999, the killing of two children, their mother and grandmother in the Welsh village of Clydach; and also in 1999, the killing by a city trader (who then killed himself) of nine office workers and his estranged wife and their two children, and the injuring of 12 others, in Atlanta, Georgia.

The term 'serial killer' also gained prominence in the 1980s (Jenkins, 1994). Fox & Levin define the phenomenon of serial killing as:

> The tendency to kill repeatedly (at least three or four victims) and often with increasing brutality, serial killers stalk their victims, one at a time, for weeks, months, or years, generally not stopping until they are caught. (Fox & Levin, 1999, p165)

For example, in 1999, Charles Ng was convicted in California of torturing and killing 11 people (men, women and children) at a mountain cabin he shared with an accomplice (who committed suicide) during the 1980s. Also in 1999, Anatoly Onoprienko, a former Ukrainian forester, admitted the murder of 52 people (10 of them children), usually using a shotgun, over a series of years and wide geographical area, mutilating some of the bodies of his victims.

The Russian serial killer Andrei Chikatilo murdered the same number of people (eating some of the bodies) and was executed in 1994. In 1999, four men were charged with Australia's largest serial killing. Eleven bodies were found in two places around Adelaide, in a garden in the suburb of Salisbury North, and packed into plastic drums inside the vault of a disused bank at Snowtown, 90 miles from the city. Again in 1999, a Kenyan serial killer, rapist and bank robber, who had previously escaped four times from prison (on the last occasion from the country's maximum security prison shortly before he was to be hanged) was rearrested. All in all, he was suspected to have committed at least 14 murders and 88 rapes, and had netted millions of pounds from his robberies. The year 2000, however, gave witness to cruelty on an unimaginable scale, with the conviction in Pakistan of Javed Iqbal, who, with accomplices, defiled and dismembered 100 children.

In England, killers who have committed murders of such abhorrence that they have been given the unusual sentence of 'whole life tariffs' include: Ian Brady and Myra Hindley, convicted of the 'Moors Murders' of a number of children in the 1960s; Donald Neilson, convicted in 1975 for a series of murders including that of the heiress Lesley Whittle; Peter Sutcliffe, given 20 life sentences in 1981 for his attacks on, and murders of, women; the nurse Beverly Allitt, who was given 13 life sentences in 1993 for injuring nine children and killing four other children in her care by smothering them or injecting insulin; and Rosemary West, convicted in 1995 of abusing and killing 10 women and children. Medical practitioner, Harold Shipman, became in 2000 England's most prolific serial killer. He was found guilty of murdering 15 of his patients and is suspected by the police of killing many more.

Killing the killers

Whilst recompense of one sort or another is invariably demanded by the state for unlawful killing, the form that the punishment takes varies considerably. Nearly a hundred countries retain the death penalty. At the end of the twentieth century, the death penalty was legal in 38 of the states of the USA (Gittings & Ellison, 1999). The USA is the only major industrialized country to preserve the act of execution for 'ordinary' murder.

In a 20-year period since the reinstatement of the death penalty in 1976, more than 500 people were executed, Texas and Virginia being the most zealous states in their use of capital punishment. At any one time, there are thousands of people waiting on 'Death Row' in the USA. For example, in 1996, it was estimated that 3000 prisoners were awaiting the outcome of protracted and multistaged appeals processes that would change their sentence, or (rarely) release them, or confirm that an execution would go ahead (Snell, 1997). The form of execution in the USA in most death penalty regions is lethal injection or the electric chair. Hanging, the gas chamber and the firing squad are also used, but by only a few states.

There is some evidence that the effect of the death penalty may be to exacerbate certain types of murder. In a study by Cochran et al. (1994), the deterrent effect of the death penalty was examined. In 1990, the State of Oklahoma, after a 25-year absence, restored capital punishment, and the first to die, amidst much media fascination, was Charles Coleman. Rates of murder, from the year previous to the execution through to the year after, were inspected by Cochran and his colleagues. The rate after the execution was not significantly higher than before. What they believed they detected, however, was a substantial rise in 'stranger' murders the week after Coleman's death compared with the week prior to his being put to death. This, they reasoned, was because of the 'brutalization' effect. That is, far from preventing further murders, the liquidation of a citizen by the state, particularly when this is widely publicized, serves to encourage (some forms) of homicide. Rather than identifying with the executed person (and thereby repressing the desire to kill for fear of the same fate), the would-be murderer takes his or her lead from the 'brutal' example of legalized killing.

Although the brutilization effect is an exceptional repercussion of legalized killing, in an overall assessment of research into the efficacy of the death penalty to prevent further homicide, William Bailey and Ruth Peterson (1999) conclude that, in general, the data do not support capital punishment being used as a deterrent for other homicides. They recommend that there needs to be a change in policy away from capital punishment in order to reduce the homicide rate. The death penalty, apart from the state reducing its expenditure by not keeping a murderer in prison perhaps for decades, and the mollification of the public's desire for retribution, seems to serve no purpose, particularly as the reoffending rate of murders is very low.

But people who are executed in the USA comprise only a fraction of those who commit offences attracting the death penalty. That is, most convicted murderers in the USA still serve jail sentences rather than being executed. China, however, is estimated to execute over 2000 of its citizens annually, and proportionally, Singapore puts to death 200 times as many of its citizens as does the USA (Gittings & Ellison, 1999). For similar crimes in most European countries, offenders will serve prison sentences rather than losing their lives (or spending much of their remaining lives on 'Death Row').

In Britain, if killing someone is classified not as murder but as manslaughter, the punishment may be a relatively short jail sentence, and, with remission for good behaviour, the period of incarceration could be cut by half. Infanticide, a common form of homicide, usually attracts in English law a relatively lenient sentence:

> A mother was jailed for three years after admitting killing her two new-born babies ... [the mother] denied murder at Leeds Crown Court, but admitted infanticide. (Unattributed news item, 1998)

But Britain, through a legal anomaly stemming from its colonial past, has retained a right to interfere with the implementation of the death penalty in other countries. In the very last year of the twentieth century, the former Caribbean colony of Trinidad and Tobago (which gained its independence in 1976) reinstated the death penalty after a five-year moratorium. However, the Privy Council's Judicial Committee of the House of Lords (functioning as the final court of appeal) had to be consulted before the hanging of a gang of nine men convicted of multiple murder could go ahead. The men, who were drug dealers, had in 1994 killed a family of four after dragging them from their beds. In June of 1999, The Judicial Committee paved the way for a backlog of 100 death sentences to be carried out by rejecting the appeal by the gang against their sentences.

In other parts of the world, punishment for killing may be modified through the acceptance of 'blood money', whereby relatives of the victim can be given financial remuneration for not insisting on the death penalty. A common form of homicide (mothers killing their own babies) is in English law considered to be a unique crime and in the main treated accordingly.

Although murder instigates a high degree of social abhorrence, this is frequently combined with unabated public fascination, as is exemplified by the plethora of books, magazines, newspaper articles and motion pictures on the subject. For example, the 1991 Hollywood film of Thomas Harris's book *Silence of the Lambs*, with Anthony Hopkins playing the murderous and cannibalistic Hannibal Lecter, was a critical and financial success, winning Academy Awards for best picture, director, actor, actress and adapted screenplay, and generating $250 million world wide. Harris's sequel to *Silence of the Lambs*, entitled simply *Hannibal*, released in 1999, was one of the biggest selling books of that year (its main competitor ironically being JK Rowling's children's book *Harry Potter and the Prisoner of Azkaban*), with a film version being prepared.

Other 'killer-thriller' films, but with even more graphic depictions of gore and death than *Silence of the Lambs* (for example, *Reservoir Dogs*, *Basic Instinct*, *Natural Born Killers* and *Seven*), have also proven popular, some achieving cult status. An investigation by the USA's Federal Trade Commission into the marketing and content of such films assessed that, by 18 years of age, American citizens would have watched on average 200 000 acts of violence and 40 000 murders on screen (Campbell, 1999).

Ironically, where films have been made about real murders, the killers themselves may be the ones to object to the commercial exploitation and public excitation of their crimes. The American serial killer David Berkowitz, serving six consecutive life sentences totalling more than 300 years, decided to give interviews to the press to voice his distress at the making of the blood-splattered scenes in the film *Summer of Sam* about his murders of young women:

> This madness, the ugliness of the past is resurfacing again: all because some people want to make some money. (Berkowitz, quoted in Harden, 1999)

Where execution is not the favoured reparation, there are examples of murderers becoming media celebrities, successful authors and stars of television programmes. In some cases, 'terrorists' who kill in the name of a cause (Zionists fighting for the creation of Israel, members of the African National Congress fighting against apartheid in South Africa, supporters of the Irish Republican Army fighting to establish a united Ireland) have become folk heroes and/or prominent politicians. Where those responsible for the illicit and deliberate killing of others have actually been executed, they have the prospect of being venerated as martyrs.

Mad murders

Establishing how many mentally disordered people commit murder is not straightforward and is not reflected in the very small number of those who acquire verdicts of 'unfit to plead' or 'not guilty by reason of insanity'. For example, from 1988 to 1997, there have been only 18 'unfit to plead' and 11 'not guilty by reason of insanity' judgements (Home Office, 1998b).

Apart from the quandary over what exactly madness is, there is much uncertainty about official statistics because of the lack of detail in traditional methods of data collection and classification. That is, these methods do not adequately expose 'madness' as a contributing or causal factor, and the final court verdict (particularly where the outcome is manslaughter) does not necessarily implicate insanity as grounds for a murderous act. Nor have the official statistics taken into account the materialization of madness in offenders after their court appearance. Furthermore, 'madness' in its broadest sense is linked to many other homicides. For example, in half of all murders, the assailant has indulged in alcohol and other forms of drug abuse. Moreover, whether the perpetrator is considered to be 'normal' or 'mad', his or her mental state immediately prior to the killing is invariably the same – intense emotional arousal. It can, therefore, be argued that virtually all murderers are mentally unstable for at least the duration of the killing.

In Britain, the DoH, in consultation with the Royal College of Psychiatrists, set up an inquiry in 1992 to grapple with the problem of identifying which murders (and suicides) could be assigned to mentally disturbed people. Home Office files were scrutinized to identify homicides in which the perpetrator had had contact with the psychiatric services or had subsequently become the responsibility of forensic psychiatry. Follow-up questionnaires were then sent to the relevant clinical team.

Over what was effectively a two-year monitoring period (July 1992 to January 1994, and September 1994 to March 1995), 39 such homicides in England and Wales were identified in what became known as the Boyd Report (Boyd, 1996). Of these, the vast majority (36) were in contact with the community psychiatric services at the time of the homicide, two still being inpatients and one having been discharged from psychiatric care within the previous year. Twenty-seven of this mentally disordered group of killers were men, and 12 women. Stabbing was the most usual method of killing (17), followed by asphyxiation. Family members were most likely to be victims. Nine women had killed their own children. Only three victims were unknown to the killer.

During the latter part of the Boyd inquiry (a period of 10 months), however, over 700 suicides by those who had used the psychiatric services were reported to the inquiry team. Well over two people per day suffering from mental illness take their own lives in England alone. The human tragedy involved in this horrific statistic is immense:

> Two years on, Patricia ... still sobs when she tells of her son, Adrian, [diagnosed as a schizophrenic] who jumped to his death from a block of flats aged 23. (Boseley, 1996)

Ignominiously for the psychiatric services, many of those who kill themselves are at the time formally detained under mental health legislation. Sube Banerjee, William Bingley and Elaine Murphy (1995) conducted a study for the Mental Health Foundation of all mental health institutions (general psychiatric units, intensive care units, secure units, special hospitals and private units) in England and Wales during the period 1992–94. They documented 206 deaths of people who were being cared for under the regulations of the 1983 Mental Health Act and whose death resulted in an inquest. Ninety-five of the cases were judged by the team (i.e. the coroner's verdict was not exclusively used) to have committed suicide, a further 10 being considered to be possible suicides or accidents. Others were considered to have died from natural causes (67), the unintended consequence of treatment (15) and accidents (13), insufficient data being available to determine the cause for the remainder. The majority of the suicides happened when the patient was on leave or had absconded, with schizophrenia the most common diagnosis.

The steering committee of the Boyd Report recognized that the calculation of the numbers of homicides and suicides attributable to mentally ill people was not comprehensive. In 1996, the work by this inquiry (funded by the government in association with the Royal College of Psychiatrists) was superseded by that of a body using new methods of data collection and a complete national sample of all homicides. The ongoing research was then to come under the directorship of Professor Louis Appleby of Manchester University. The Home Office now notifies the inquiry team of any murder, manslaughter or infanticide convictions. Any psychiatric reports available from the case or previous offences are then obtained. Where the perpetrator has at any time in the past been in contact with the mental health services, questionnaires are sent to the individual consultant psychiatrists who had provided treatment.

A progress report was published one year after the commencement of the research. From a sample of 238 convictions for homicide, 17% ($n = 39$) were reported to have had symptoms of mental illness (delusions, hallucinations and depression). A further 26% ($n = 62$) had had other types of mental disorder (alcohol and drug dependence, and personality disorder) at the time of the offence (Appleby, 1997).

In 1999, more findings from this research were produced, covering an 18 consecutive case period after April 1996 (Appleby, 1999). Of the 718 convictions for homicide, 14% ($n = 102$) had had contact with the mental health services at some stage in their lives, and in 8% ($n = 58$) of these, the contact had been within the previous year. Psychiatric reports were available for 500 (70%) of the total homicide group. From this sample, symptoms of mental illness (delusions, hallucinations or depression) were noted in 71 (14%) cases. This group was less likely to kill strangers than those not recorded as suffering from symptoms of mentally illness. Using the same sample, evidence of mental disorder (defined as mental illness, personality disorder or alcohol and drug dependence) at any point in the lifetime of the perpetrator existed in 220 cases (44%). This represented 31% of the total number of homicides.

The tally of mentally disordered homicides in the findings from Appleby (1999) remains inconclusive as it excludes those people who are suspected of a killing but who commit suicide before conviction, and those who are either unfit to plead or who are found not guilty by reason of insanity. For the 18 months covered, these exemptions totalled 56, the vast majority of whom ($n = 49$) were suicides. Moreover, the inquiry team conceded that the figures for those who had a previous psychiatric history were underestimates. It is likely that some contacts were not uncovered, for example because of inadequate record keeping by mental health service personnel.

Once again, however, the research by Appleby (1999) and his team points out the discrepancy between homicide and suicide by mentally disordered people. Nearly a quarter of all suicides ($n = 1000$) are committed by people who had been in contact with the mental health services within the year before their death.

Taylor & Gunn (1999), in their analysis of the number of convictions of manslaughter on the grounds of diminished responsibility, infanticide and verdicts of 'not guilty by reason of insanity' and 'unfit to plead', conclude that the proportion of homicides attributable to the mentally disordered has declined annually by 3%. This percentage, however, does not include the scores of murder suspects who commit suicide prior to trial, many (if not all) of whom could be considered *ipso facto* to be suffering from some form of psychological distress. Without the latter group, the figures supplied by Taylor & Gunn indicate a mean average of 83 murders by mentally disordered people each year during the period 1957–95, with the highest number (130) in 1972 and lowest (41) in 1957.

Michael Howlett (1998) argues that there is a growing number of researchers who now accept that there is a correlation between violence and mental illness. Studies from a number of countries, he records, indicate that people suffering from schizophrenia are more likely than the non-mentally disordered to arm themselves and commit acts of violence and homicide as a result of their delusions. He quotes, for example, a study by Eronen et al. (1996) of 1423 homicides perpetrated over a 12-year period in Finland. These researchers found that men with a primary diagnosis of schizophrenia were six times, and women five times, more likely to kill than the respective gender in the general population.

Summary

As with all social 'facts', there are degrees of interpretation that have to be taken into account before we can be sure about what is meant by 'homicide'. However, the moral dilemma associated with warfare and capital punishment, and the apparent condoning by the state of killing 'in certain circumstances', should not detract from the gravity of 'civil' murder. Homicide is a presiding and perpetual social problem. Moreover, although we cannot be certain of the exact number of mentally disordered people who are involved in this social problem, this should not lead to the conclusion that their role is inconsequential.

Chapter 4
Faulty individuals

The concepts of crime, madness and homicide have been discussed broadly in the preceding three chapters. In the next four chapters, a series of theoretical genres will be applied to the subject of criminality, with either immediate or oblique relevance to murder and madness.

The first of these theoretical genres encompasses a number of different strands, all of which – in one way or another – regard crime and deviancy as being fixed in the make-up (biological and/or psychological) of the person conducting the infringement. It is in the individual that 'fault' is to be found, either because that person is wilfully malevolent, or because his or her evolutionary antecedents and biochemical compounds operate as impelling forces. Hence, within this framework, the 'facts' of crime and deviancy can be analysed and be seen to determine (criminal and deviant) behaviour. Moreover, science is expected to find solutions to crime and deviancy.

Social contract

The seventeenth century saw the gestation and flourishing of libertarian ideas. Libertarianism fundamentally altered the conceptualization of human 'nature' and how criminals were treated by the state. The legal processes in the Middle Ages had been unregulated, putrescent, capricious and dispassionate. They embraced all manner of imprecise categories of misdemeanour, including madness, vagrancy and 'immorality', within their scope. The central doctrine within the new philosophies decreed that humans were rational', free to make their own choices, but hedonistic. All humans, therefore, in their drive to secure pleasure and avoid pain, had the potential to commit crime.

Classical criminology, taking its lead from these ideas, saw the egotistical forces of humans balanced with a consensual drive from society as a whole to have the extremes that emerged from self-interest modified by the law. Moreover, the medieval notion that criminals were possessed by demons, and that both rights, and the type and level of atonement, depended on the social status of the individual, was displaced. The specific behaviours of the individual were now targeted for punishment. However, unlike what occurred in the Middle Ages (where being found guilty of what today we would consider to be minor offences might have resulted in execution), the punishment should fit the crime.

Consequently, in order that individual citizens and their properties were safeguarded, a 'contract', representing the needs of the individual and those of the community, was enforced by a 'just' legal system that dispensed 'fair' punishments.

Jean-Jacques Rousseau (1712–1778) based his philosophical work *Du Contrat Social* on the premise that the 'perfect nature of man' could be defiled by a corrupt society. Rousseau was also to influence the drawing-up of the 1787 American Constitution and the 1789 French revolutionaries' declaration of 'The Rights of Man'. For Rousseau, society had to be ordered in such a way as to ensure that corruption was at a minimum, and that each person would therefore be more amenable to contributing to the overall good of society:

> the social order is a sacred right which is the basis of all other rights ... The problem is to find a form of association which will defend and protect with the whole common force the person and goods of each associate, and in which each, while uniting himself with all, may still obey himself alone, and remain as free as before. (Rousseau, 1762, p174)

So, the libertarians and classicist criminologists viewed individuals as willingly entering into, in Rousseau's terms, a 'form of association' that had the mutual benefit of protecting all participants in this association as well as the social system overall. It was the individual's duty to act within, and to uphold, the law. The responsibility of the state was to rectify recalcitrance by using punishments that equated with the severity of the crime. The assessment of humans as rational and operating with free will resulted in the law operating from the position that all before it should be treated equally, and hence mitigating circumstances were inapplicable as a form of defence (Taylor et al., 1981). Intent, motivation, speculation about cause, and social disadvantage were not taken into account when sentence was passed.

The social contract, however, was a 'social control' covenant that, although appearing to condone equality, in effect supported the ideology and interests of the rising bourgeois class. That is, individualism, personal achievement and the ownership of property were sanctioned implicitly by the social contract (Gouldner, 1971). Hence, under the social contract, there was to be no readjustment of the structural inequalities that had been created by the inheritance and acquisition of property. Indeed, property was construed as being the essence of progressive (i.e. bourgeois) 'civil society':

> It is certain that the right of property is the most sacred of all the rights of citizenship, and even more important in some respects than liberty itself; either because it more nearly affects the preservation of life, or because, property being more easily usurped and more difficult to defend than life, the law ought to pay a greater attention to what is more easily taken away; or finally, because property is the true foundation of civil society, and the real guarantee of the undertakings of citizens. (Rousseau, 1762, p138)

However, whereas such philosophers as Rousseau gave importance to the centrality of property within the developing capitalist mode of economic production, this was not without some recognition of the tension between 'ownership' and social strife. In the following passage, Rousseau refers to the paradox of the Enlightenment for what he terms 'civil society'. The settlement and expropriation of land was also to be the source of untold human tribulation:

> The first man who, having enclosed a piece of ground, bethought himself of saying 'This is Mine', and found people simple enough to believe him, was the real founder of civil society. From how many crimes, wars, and murders, from how many horrors and misfortunes might not any one have saved mankind, by pulling up his stakes, or filling up his ditch, and crying to his fellows: 'Beware of listening to this impostor; you are undone if you once forget that the fruits of the earth belong to us all, and the earth itself to nobody'. (Rousseau, 1762, p76)

For Rousseau, it is the role of the law to mediate between the consequences of avarice and the 'common good' in a propertied society. In practice, however, the beneficiaries of any preservation of the 'common good' belonged to a stratum of society with a vested interest in maintaining the social order, and people at the bottom of the social hierarchy (i.e. those without estate) had their structural disadvantage compounded by laws based on an equal distribution of punishment.

Eventually, modifications had to be made to laws that in general ignored prevailing beliefs about human nature and dismissed widespread experiences of poverty, disease and social discrimination, as well as the personal failings and attributes of the offender. That is, the purity of the classicist conception of humanity as rational and containing isolated individuals who were wholly responsible for their own actions was tempered with a limited acknowledgement of various social situations that can shape behaviour. Thus, the neo-classicists:

> took the solitary rational man of classicist criminology and gave him a past and a future. With an eye to the influence of factors which might determine the commission of a criminal act and the actions of a man subsequent to conviction, they held fast to the notion of human volition. They merely sketched in the structures which might blur or marginally affect the exercise of voluntarism. (Taylor et al., 1981, p9)

The key characteristics of the version of social contract theory emanating from neo-classicism are described by Taylor et al. (1981):

1. Individuals remain accountable for their actions, but the circumstances of the accused can be taken into account for the purpose of 'mitigation'; they cannot, however, be used to excuse criminal behaviour.
2. There is an acceptance of the need to adjust the level and type of punishment in order to allow for the possibility of rehabilitation.
3. Some sections of society (the very young and the elderly) may not be held fully accountable for their decisions.
4. Certain other groups of individuals can be exonerated of responsibility for their behaviour on the basis that they are inherently 'irrational' (principally, those classified as 'feeble-minded' or 'mad').

5. Expert opinion from disciplines other than that of the legal
    profession (e.g. psychiatry) enters the arena of the court.
6. The imperative to have sentences 'fit the crime' is to some
    degree assuaged. (For example, it becomes more probable that
    those deemed mentally retarded or insane will be given punish-
    ments different from those meted out to those deemed intellec-
    tually and psychologically lucid.)

The refashioned classicist perception of the social contract has,
in one form or another, persisted into the twentieth century. Indeed,
re-creating the social contract became part of a late twentieth-
century political discourse throughout the industrialized world,
particularly in Europe and the USA. It was even projected as paramount in the re-forming of the 'special relationship' between the
USA and Britain:

> Sydney Blumenthal ... one of President Clinton's close advisors ... told a
> meeting of the World Policy Institute: 'With Great Britain we have forged a
> new special relationship, a 21st century alliance, as the President [Clinton]
> called it, based not only on all our traditional mutual interests but on our
> common conviction of the necessity for a *new social contract*.' (Castle &
> Usborne, 1998, emphasis added).

The Britain of the 1980s saw the political rhetoric of the 'new
right' being directed towards what was perceived to be a 'form of
association' in which there was too much state control over both
industry and the citizen's everyday life. The pendulum, argued political theorists of this radical persuasion, had swung too far in favour
of interference at the level of the economic, social and personal.
Famously, Margaret Thatcher, the British Conservative Prime
Minister from 1979 to 1989, announced that there was no such
entity as 'society'. Under her influence, and that of her successor
John Major, policies were installed to re-establish an atomized, self-
possessed and empowered citizen. The 'common good' became
equated with individual success.

The political messages of the British 'New Labour' government,
elected in 1997 under the leadership of Tony Blair, once again,
however, make explicit the bond that individuals have with the
community. The Labour government's search for a 'Third Way' in

British politics, which mediates between the individualism of rampant monetarist economics and the social engineering of the 'nanny state', has entered all areas of social policy, including that of education, crime and health. For example, this government was to argue that the state education system should encourage individuals to accept the moral obligations of citizenship, as well as such specific duties as 'parenting' (Carvel, 1998; Walker, 1998).

Professor Anthony Giddens, in his book *The Third Way: The Renewal of Social Democracy* (1998), observes that there have been fundamental changes in world politics and economics (principally caused by globalisation) that demand new social agreements. Using slogans such as 'No authority without democracy' and 'No rights without responsibilities', Giddens argues that there is a need for all those in society (workers, employers and government) to form an alliance in order to 'help citizens pilot their way through the major revolutions of our time' (Giddens, 1998, p64).

For Giddens, regenerating community life and 'civility' will help to prevent crime and reduce the public's fear of crime. Therefore, there must be a shift from law enforcement to crime prevention policies by the police, and the creation of an all-embracing network of partnerships aimed at reducing urban decay, which then will assist in the re-establishment of civil order, increase the quality of life and improve social justice:

> In order to work, partnerships between government agencies, the criminal justice system, local associations and community organisations have to be inclusive – all economic and ethnic groups must be involved. Government and business can act together to help repair urban decay. (Giddens, 1998, p88)

There is, however, something quite naive about furthering the cause of unity in a society riddled with rivalries and disparity. Moreover, a social contract based on the political soundbite 'Partnership for prosperity' masks the fact that it is only one section of society that ultimately gains from social cohesion:

> Everyone cannot be a winner – the tobacco and health lobbies, for example, cannot both win – and there will always be losers ... this new civic partnership requires the poor to get a job, go back to college, clean up their estate, run Neighbourhood Watch, and so on. But what was it big business had to

> do again? You look back through [Gidden's book], and find that business
> must be rewarded with generous tax breaks for participating in new Third
> way initiatives. When Giddens and Blair talk about 'what works' they
> primarily mean 'what works for business'. (Aitkenhead, 1998).

Accepting, however, that those at the bottom of the social hierarchy suffer much more from most of the major causes of premature
death than those who belong to the higher classes, the Blair government has targeted both social structure and individual behaviour
(Department of Health, 1999d). That is, the new contract involves,
on the one hand, citizens adopting preventative measures (eating
healthy food, taking regular exercise, practising 'safe sex', giving up
smoking, not abusing drugs and drinking alcohol in moderation),
and on the other, the government tackling the issues of 'social exclusion' (poverty, unemployment and homelessness) and poor environmental conditions (pollution, danger in the workplace and
overcrowded living conditions).

Positivism

By the nineteenth century, 'positivistic' science was offered as the
sole and legitimate exegetic paradigm for both the physical and the
social world. Gerard Delanty (1997) has catalogued the core tenets
of positivism. These include the following:

1.   All knowledge is susceptible to the techniques of natural science.
2.   'Scienticism' – only scientific knowledge is credible.
3.   There is a reality that can be studied, and science stands ('objec-
     tively' and value-free) outside this reality.
4.   Empiricism – we only know what can be observed, and the
     experiment is the basis of scientific observation.
5.   Internally coherent and universal laws exist that cross over
     bodies of knowledge and accord with the properties of reality.

So, for the positivist social scientist, society can be studied using
the same principles and procedures as physics, chemistry and mathematics. There are, argues the positivist, cause and effect relationships
between social phenomena. Just as mathematical formulae and the
laws of physics allow us to predict how a car or rocket will perform,

the science of sociology and anthropology can identify the origins of 'the family' and anticipate future patterns in human consanguinity.

As with other disciplines involved in the study of human behaviour, criminology has been affected by scientific positivism. The consequence of this has been to steer the study of crime in the direction of attempting to find causality, the measurement of criminality, and social policies aimed at control (Walklate, 1998). Moreover, the mission of the positivist school of criminology is the complete eradication of antisocial behaviour. The locus of criminological study is destined to become biology and evolution. Criminals, positivistic criminology posits, act in the way in which they do because they have no choice: their molecular disposition propels them towards irresponsibility.

Some medical practitioners of the nineteenth century, adopting the principles of positivism, saw what they believed to be an affiliation between criminality and mental disorder. That is, crime and madness could be viewed as a unified and congenitally created 'caste'. Dr Thomson of the General Prison in Perth, Scotland, studying his population of 'intractable' and 'inter-generational' prisoners, came to a five-point conclusion:

1. That there is a *criminal class* distinct from other civilised and criminal men.
2. That this criminal class is marked by peculiar physical and mental characteristics.
3. That the hereditary nature of crime is seen by the *family* histories of criminals.
4. That the *transformation* of other nervous disorders with crime in the criminal class, also proves the alliance of hereditary crime with other disorders of the mind – such as epilepsy, dipsomania, insanity, etc.
5. That the *incurable* nature of crime in the criminal class goes to prove its hereditary nature. (Thomson, 1870, p488, original emphases).

One prevailing idea from the positivist school of the nineteenth century was that of 'atavism'. Following Darwin's postulations about evolutionary development, the anthropological criminologist Cesare

Lombroso (1876) argued that 'normal' humans during their life-time experience all of the stages that the species has undergone in its process of evolution. Abnormal behaviour was thus a 'throw-back' to a previous primitive juncture in the history of humankind. For the biological positivist, atavism could be observed in individual physiognomy (sloping foreheads, an oversized jaw and cheek bones, protruding ears, oversized arms, large orbital cavities, abnormal genitalia, excessive hairiness and extra toes, fingers and nipples) and in certain extreme habits (excessive indolence, tattooing and a love of orgies).

The belief that physiognomic characteristics could indicate social maladjustment was later extended to the whole body. For example, William Sheldon (1949) suggested that the human corporeality could be divided into three types: (a) the mesomorph (muscular, well-proportioned and physically active); (b) the ectomorph (with a thin physical build); and (c) the endomorph (rotund and slothful). Delinquents, it was postulated, were much more likely to be mesomorphs.

In the 1820s and 30s, the homicidally insane were accredited by some American and British alienists, not with external physiognomic abnormality, but with intracranial peculiarities based on the phrenological observations of Franz Joseph Gall. The 'science' of phrenology propounded the view that the brain could be mapped showing discrete anatomical organs of human mental functioning and behaviour, such as hope, spirituality, self-esteem, parental love, combativeness, benevolence, veneration, firmness and conscientiousness. Gall believed, on the evidence of an examination of the brains of two murderers, that there was also a localized 'Organ of Murder' to be found above the ear (Colaizzi, 1989). In the brains of killers, this organ was enlarged.

Lombroso's theory of 'wrong-headedness' gave much sustenance to somatic psychiatry in the later parts of the nineteenth and the early part of the twentieth century. But atavism as such has been discredited on the basis that the statistical methods used to assess the incidence of evolutionary degeneration and its association with deviancy were unreliable. Moreover, physiognomical irregularities attract social stigma and the attention of law enforcers, thereby creating the possibility of a 'self-fulfilling prophecy' (Taylor et al., 1981).

However, although atavism in the form proposed by Lombroso is no longer plausible, biological explanations for 'bad conduct' are today flourishing (Laurance, 1998). New brain scanning and imaging technologies, experimentation into the functioning of neurochemicals such as dopamine and serotonin, and genetic mapping are underscoring the premises of positivism and biological determinism.

Neo-Darwinianism

'Boys are made to squirt and girls are made to lay eggs. And if the truth be known, boys don't very much care what they squirt into'. Crude though it may be, Gore Vidal's pithy quote neatly sums up the argument for evolutionary psychology. (Malik, 1998, p1)

The upsurge of interest in evolution has been embraced fervently by psychology (Brannigan, 1997; Nicholson, 1997) and has gained converts in psychiatry (Stevens & Price, 1996; McGuire & Troisi, 1998). Modern evolutionary theory, applied to social development and human nature, has, however, gone beyond the raw reductionist premise of 'survival of the fittest' and the 'selfish gene'. The individual not only strives to maintain his or her own existence (either through direct self-protection measures or by ensuring that his or her genes endure), and in this process is acquisitive and competitive, but also collaborates with others in order to achieve personal goals. That is, there exists in the human condition both selfishness and 'reciprocal altruism'.

Peter Singer, director of the Centre for Human Biothetics at Monash University, describes the predicament of individuals when they have to decide whether or not to cooperate (the so-called 'prisoner dilemma'):

The prisoner dilemma describes a situation in which two people can each choose whether or not to cooperate with each other. The catch is that each does better, individually, by not cooperating; but if both make this choice, they will be both worse off than they would have been if they had not pursued their own interest. The individual pursuit of self-interest can be collectively self-defeating. (Singer, 1998, p29).

Singer goes on to illustrate how many of us have to contend daily with a version of the 'prisoner dilemma'. When travelling to work by

car, we are participating in behaviours that affect detrimentally
fellow commuters and the community at large. That is, we help to
create traffic jams, pollute the environment and collude with others
in an inefficient method of conveying people from home to their
place of employment. If we were to make the decision to use public
transport, the road would be less congested and the air cleaner.
However, not only do we wish that all of our fellow car drivers would
use buses and trains so that our journey by car would be made easier,
but we also recognize that unless a substantial number of commuters
switch to public transport, there will be little investment in these
services to make them a suitable alternative. We are all, therefore,
caught in a trap of waiting for the other person to make the move.

Research into cooperative behaviour by Robert Axelrod (1984)
has indicated that there is a 'tit-for-tat' phenomenon. That is,
humans are inclined to initiate and repay selfless behaviour in kind
because there is an inherent appreciation of collaboration being ultimately advantageous to them. However, if the other person defaults
on this pro-social expectation, we may also stop our cooperative
behaviour. Put simply, if asked, we are likely to give our neighbour a
bowl of sugar if he or she has offered us the same service in the past
because we implicitly foresee a time in the future when we might
need another favour. We are disinclined to provide a neighbour with
food (or anything else) if on a previous occasion our request for help
has been responded to negatively – in evolutionary terms, there is no
advantage for us personally to do so.

It has been argued, however, that the 'pay-off' for cooperating
with others becomes less feasible in social configurations in which
individuals have little chance of reconnecting at some prospective
point in time:

> Tit for Tat cannot work in a society of strangers who will never encounter
> each other again. This is why people living in big cities do not always show
> consideration to each other that is the norm in rural villages in which people
> have known each other all their lives. (Singer, 1998, p30)

If individuals do not enter gratuitously into 'helping' each other
because certain social structures precipitate anticooperative behaviours, deviancy and crime may be the consequence. That is, social
organizations (or even whole societies) that are alienating in their

effect will produce individuals who will challenge society and its institutions through their non-cooperative actions. As Singer points out, if people are marginalized (through poverty, unemployment or incarceration in prisons or psychiatric establishments) and do not participate in mainstream social activities, they will have no reason to invest personally in the social values of their community.

Research by the zoologist Martin Nowak and the mathematician Karl Sigmund (1998) has, however, added a new dimension to the understanding of cooperation by suggesting that there are, in evolutionary terms, pay-offs for 'being nice' to others even if there is no obvious possibility of any reciprocal gesture. Equally, they argue that 'being mean' is likely to lead to evolutionary failure. Random, unconditional acts of magnanimity are rewarded indirectly as the 'givers' benefit from the goodwill of the community.

Transnational studies of twins have indicated familial links with crime. In these studies, identical twins were much more likely to have criminal records than non-identical twins (Raine, 1993). In addition, research into adopted children with natural parents who were criminals has suggested that these children had a higher rate of criminality than adopted children whose parents did not have criminal records (Raine, 1993).

The case of Russell Grant-McVicar illustrates well the biological determinist claim of the link between inherited genes and behaviour. Russell Grant-McVicar, the son of John McVicar, who served a life sentence after being convicted of armed robbery in the 1960s, was himself jailed in 1998 for a series of armed robberies, which included the theft of a Picasso painting:

> The 12-day trial had heard how Grant-McVicar seized the Picasso, Tête de Femme ... after storming into the Lefevre gallery in Mayfair, central London, and opening a holdall to reveal a double-barrelled shotgun. When a member of staff refused to hand over the Picasso, he wrenched it from the wall and pointing the gun at a cab driver who was waiting for him, fled to south London. (Hall, 1998a)

The biological evidence here appears to be strong – the son of a violent man, who is reported to have had only a limited association with his father during his childhood, is convicted of crimes that involve the threat of violence.

On the other hand, Clinard & Meier (1995) point out that, despite the long history of 'positivism' within criminology, the exact molecular and chemical mechanisms that direct behavioural pathology in humans have not been found. Significantly, they highlight the difficulty in accepting the 'biological imperative' when criminal and deviant behaviour is defined by laws and social norms that can change over relatively short periods of time and in different social circumstances. Not only can some categories of 'normality' become reclassified as criminal (as has been the case of driving whilst under the influence of alcohol), but also some acts (for example, homosexuality) can move their status from 'criminal' to be accepted as part of 'normal' behaviour.

Furthermore, for Russell Grant-McVicar, restricted primary socialization with his father does not necessarily mean that biology caused his criminality: other socio-environmental influences might have been at work. No doubt McVicar junior was aware of McVicar senior's reputation through, for example, the media, and he may well have consciously attempted to emulate (or even spite) his father. Moreover, any biologically determined urge to commit crime seems to have abated in John McVicar himself. Notwithstanding his former reputation as 'Britain's public enemy No.1' in the 1960s (and being cleared of causing actual bodily harm in an argument with a neighbour in the 1990s), he became famous as a 'reformed criminal', obtained two university degrees and became a broadcaster and an author (Hall, 1998b).

The reaction of some social scientists to the growing popularization of evolutionary and biological explanations of human behaviour can be interpreted as being nakedly partisan and protectionist. For example, although Tom Shakespeare calls for sociologists to attend to human corporeity, he is emphatic in his hostility to what he describes as the 'new biologism', and argues for intellectual battle lines to be drawn up in order to defend the credibility and praxis of social theory:

> it is an intellectual imperative to demolish the shaky constructions which the new biologism has advanced: we [sociologists] cannot ignore spurious misrepresentations of causality and the social world ... evolutionary psychology and neurogenetic determinism are an explicit threat to the professional practice of sociology as a discipline: we need to look to our borders and our claim to explanatory competence. (Shakespeare, 1997, p32)

Combination theory

Yet there are signs that purists from both the DNA-centric and social-deterministic camps can benefit from an approach to Darwinian 'natural selection' that accepts the influence of culture on the evolutionary destiny of humanity. 'Gene-culture co-evolutionary theory' challenges Richard Dawkins' (1989) claim that the catalyst for the shaping of human development is not at the level of society, social groupings or even the organism itself. For Dawkins, humans are impelled by the smallest element of life – the gene. Humans as totalities, therefore, are construed as passively interreacting with their physical and social environment. It is the gene which struggles to adapt to external pressures.

However, Steven Rose (1997), Professor of Biology at the Open University, argues that Dawkins' 'genetic imperialism' fails to acknowledge the ways in which environments are chosen by organisms and subsequently altered by the culture of these organisms. The proponents of gene-culture co-evolutionary theory argue that the interplay between culture and genes is complex and reflexive. It is accepted that the genetic make-up of the human organism will affect the manifestation of culture. However, it is suggested that some cultural practices change the environment, and these changes in living conditions then serve to influence the selection of particular genes. As Laura Spinney notes, culture and genetics become 'twin driving forces in directing the evolutionary pathway' (1997, p28).

Research into left-handedness provides an illustration of how cultural practices and genes work conjointly to produce evolutionary modifications. As Robert Mathews (1997) records, gene-culture co-evolutionary theorists, using sophisticated mathematical models, have found that knowing whether people are right-handed or left-handed does not help in knowing which hand will be preferred by their siblings, and this is the case even for identical twins. However, the social environment does appear to impact on which hand becomes dominant. There are historical changes in the rates of left-handedness in the same country, as well as disparate rates of left-handedness in different countries. In North America in the nineteenth century, only about 2% of the population were left-handed, but the rate in the late twentieth century became almost 12%. In Taiwan, the rate remains less than 1%. What the findings from this research imply is that there is a genetic predilection towards right-handedness but that cultural norms may encourage parents to influence which hand the child eventually prefers to use.

Gene-culture co-evolutionary theory is also being utilized to link cultural preferences to the skewed sex ratio in favour of a greater number of male births. The work of Kevin Laland of Cambridge University, and Jochen Kumm and Marcus Feldman of Stanford University, indicates that the higher socio-economic status of males in comparison with females may have led to a sex-biased birth rate:

> Parents who were genetically more likely to produce daughters ended up killing more of their children, steadily reducing their representation in the gene pool relative to parents predisposed to have sons. So this bias towards male births may be a grim echo of past female infanticide. (Mathews, 1997, p31)

Evolutionary violence

Daly & Wilson (1999) point out that homicides are not indiscriminate events. From their analysis of who kills and who gets killed, they have produced what they describe as 'conflict typologies' concerning the relationship between the victim and the killer. That is, homicides are, for Daly & Wilson, invariably about young men attempting to gain dominance over each other, women attempting to gain independence from proprietary partners or ex-partners, and the disposing of children by those entrusted with their care. Evolutionary psychology, Daly & Wilson suggest, can help to explain these patterns.

Interestingly, Daly & Wilson postulate that violence is not necessarily a pathological behaviour. Humans, along with many other animals, are designed to deal with, and enact, violence. This they do for self-protection and to survive in situations where resources and breeding opportunities are scarce. Challenging the structural theories of crime (which are predicated on such factors as economic disparity, and social strain and disorganization), Daly & Wilson argue that, in some societies (for example, tribal communities), it is those at the top of the social hierarchy who are the most violent. Here violence is used to maintain dominance for an élite and stability for the community, rather than as a reaction by the disempowered to social inequality and decay.

Although not wishing to posit that homicide is intrinsically an evolved behaviour, enabling humans to adapt to their environment, Daly & Wilson claim that violence is functional to self-interest. However, they do provide an evolutionary explanation for the common types of murder. For example, they argue that the presence of step-parents in 'reconstituted' families poses an important risk factor in child abuse and killings as the result of an imbalance in the investment/benefit ratio. That is, unlike the case with biological parents, step-parents have no genetic pay-off for their material and emotional input into the rearing of dependent children.

Moreover, for the evolutionist, homicide between sexual partners is more likely when there is evidence or suspicion of infidelity. This is especially the case when it is the woman who has been seen by the man to have undermined his genetic potential by engaging in sexual activity with other men.

Men killing unrelated men is also tackled by Daly & Wilson's evolutionary theorizing. This occurs, they suggest, quite simply because of the evolutionary drive of 'competition' between men. That is, murder may be the outcome of contests concerning money and other material possessions, sexual partners or social status. These conflicts may be immediate or long term. For example, a fatality may be the result of a 'spontaneous' night-club brawl between men over a prospective girlfriend. On the hand, the higher rate of homicide amongst people at the lower end of the social system may be grounded in feelings of retribution aimed at an unfair society.

Unrefined evolutionary theorizing is unconvincing, however, primarily because it is teleological and reductionist. Biological reductionism cannot explain the wide variety of human behaviour and differences in cultural practices. As Steven Rose argues, fallacious claims over such issues as criminality and homicide are made by the evolutionary theorists:

> Crimes of violence are more frequently carried out by men than women ... One may argue that this says something about the Y chromosome, carried by men and not women, but the overwhelming majority of men are not violent criminals ... Violent crime is much higher in the USA than in Europe – higher, for instance than in Britain, and much higher than in Sweden. Could this be accounted for by some unique feature of the American geno-

type? Well, possibly, but pretty unlikely, since much of the American population originated by migration from Europe. But also the rates of violent
crime change dramatically over quite short time periods. (Rose, 1997, p298)

Rose observes that a key factor in the USA homicide rate is not
evolutionary genetic drives but the estimated 280 million hand guns
in the personal possession of its citizens.

Medical science

The profession of medicine has an inexorable link with scientific
positivism. The positivistic underpinnings of the natural sciences
and technology have been used by medicine as 'ideological ammuni-
tion' in the process of professionalization (Morgan et al., 1985;
Morrall, 1998). That is, medicine 'rides on the back' of - as well as
contributing to - the proclaimed successes of science, and has
thereby achieved the status of a pre-eminent occupation. The institution of medicine, with science as its epistemological benefactor,
individuates social problems through the process of medicalization,
and thereby serves as a major agency of control:

> The medicalisation of deviance, and attendant medical social control, is
> becoming increasingly prevalent in modern industrial societies. (Conrad,
> 1981, p102)

Medicine, as a proactive and imperialistic enterprise, continues
to colonize new areas of work. Each year, a multitude of novel
diseases are 'discovered': repetitive strain injury, complete mass
conflict disorder, false memory syndrome, Munchausen's by proxy,
jogger's nipple, knitter's finger, Chinese restaurant syndrome. The
course of how a woman's state of mind prior to menstruation
became a fully fledged psychosomatic affliction is charted by Cather-
ine Bennett:

> Menstruation always did have a scurvy reputation, what with blighting crops
> and souring milk, but it took 20th century science to discover that women
> could be possessed by evil spirits before their periods had even begun. In
> 1931, pre-menstrual days were found to be a time of tension and hostility.
> They deserved a name of their own: PMT [premenstrual tension]. In 1953
> Dr Katharina Dalton ... spotted a multitude of new symptoms, and invented
> something better: Pre-menstrual Syndrome, or PMS. This majestical
> syndrome embraces clumsiness, amnesia, fatigue, depression, anxiety,

mood-swings – 150 different symptoms! It can account for completely differ-
ent states of mind: lethargic and energetic; lecherous and unresponsive ...
PMS has been accepted as an excuse for shoplifiting, arson and homicide.
(Bennett, 1993)

Medical practitioner James Le Fanu points out that a huge
number of people are diagnosed as having what he describes as 'non-
diseases', and that this is a growing phenomenon due principally to
the expansion of health screening. For example, he argues that tens
of thousands are classified as 'hypertensive', and are prescribed
medication on that basis, as a result of a doctor at some time taking
their blood pressure as part of a formal or *ad hoc* assessment of
general health. He even suggests that a minority of women have
been erroneously diagnosed as having breast cancer because a
'lump' has been detected and pathologists are likely to want to err on
the side of caution. However, these women continue throughout
their lives to suffer from the psychological distress that this diagnosis
entails, let alone the bodily disfigurement of any resultant radiologi-
cal or surgical treatment. Le Fanu goes on to identify what he
believes to be the most prevalent way in which non-diseases are
concocted:

Much the commonest sources of non-disease today are the routine biochemical tests to measure the level of chemicals such as uric acid or cholesterol in
the blood or to assess the functioning of the thyroid gland. Back comes an
'abnormal' result from the lab and, hey presto, someone who is well
suddenly acquires a non-disease such as myxoedema (an under-active
thyroid) or hypercholesteraemia (excess of cholesterol) requiring medication
for life. (Le Fanu, 1997)

Medicine is not, however, mandated solely by science and technology (Seedhouse, 1991). There are very different forms of knowledge and treatment across and within the various medical
specialisms: the trade of psychiatry cannot easily be compared with
that of microsurgery, for example. Moreover, as Anthony Clare
(1976) has observed, psychiatry is eclectic. The interventions of
cognitive-behavioural therapy and the psychopharmacological
effects of antidepressant or antipsychotic chemicals have minimal
epistemological synchronicity. Put another way, the history of psychiatry is made up of contending lore and policy. Asylumdom has

competed with care in the community, psychoanalysis and 'moral therapy' with the artefacts of somatic medicine.

But medicine is ultimately and vitally swayed by science, and scientific measurement and validation are projected as being the ideal. Furthermore, medical practice has been seduced by an 'epidemic of techno-scientific discovery' that has taken place in the last quarter of the twentieth century (Nuland, 1996). There have been revolutionary advances taking place in physics, chemistry, mathematics, computer technology, molecular and cell biology, and pharmacology, all of which medicine has devoured and proclaimed as its own.

The medical profession, even with the aid of a flourishing science, has, however, still not conquered heart attacks, strokes, AIDS or even the common cold (Weatherall, 1995). Despite improvements in treatment, the number of diabetes and asthma sufferers continues to grow, antibiotics are beginning to be considered a scourge because they are reducing the resistance of the population as a whole to disease, and pulmonary tuberculosis, malaria and cholera remain endemic in many parts of the world. Moreover, the health of the poor in the industrialized world, although improved overall, has become worse relative to that of the rich, as has the health of the majority in developing countries compared with that of Western populations.

Furthermore, not only is medicine lagging behind the reality of its own propaganda, but also the iatrogenic consequences of its interventions are potent and widespread. Abraham (1995), for example, suggests that the testing and regulation of pharmaceutical products remains far from satisfactory. Abraham points out that the public is perpetually at risk from such medical catastrophes as the 'thalidomide incident', whereby pregnant women were given a 'safe' drug, which was then found to cause severe foetal deformities. The editor of *The Lancet*, Richard Horton, gives warning that:

> drugs are licensed by government and marketed by industry well before they are proved safe. An alarmist claim? Only last month, Troglitazine, a drug launched in October [1997] and prescribed to 5,000 British diabetics (and with world sales of $137 million) was withdrawn from the UK by Glaxo Wellcome because it was worried about damaging side effects on the liver. (Horton, 1998)

Professor Richard Smith, Editor of the *British Medical Journal*, in a report of his speech at an annual conference of the Royal College of Psychiatrists (Boseley, 1998a), has acknowledged the poor quality of medical knowledge. He has argued that, at best, only 5% of articles in all of the twenty thousand published medical journals around the world have any scientific merit or application to clinical practice. The results of studies reported in these journals are often contradictory, biased and ungeneralizable, and some may also be fraudulent. Smith has suggested that the empirically driven policy of the British government for 'evidence-based medicine', aimed at improving treatment, will inevitably falter unless standards in research improve.

These deficiencies in the practice of medicine are, however, counterbalanced by the well-publicized promise of future accomplishments that the new techno-scientific knowledge offers. Coinciding with reports of medical malpractice and ineffectiveness, stories abound in the popular media (and academic journals) of how medical genetics and pharmacology are providing new cures for cancer, coronary failure and senile dementia, as well as having the potential to prevent inherited defects.

For example, in the same edition of the *Guardian* newspaper, the following two contrasting articles about medical competency/incompetency were published. The first was a lengthy account of one month's spate of media stories about 'disgraced' doctors, and ran with the headline 'Bad medicine':

> What has happened to our doctors, those men and women with stethoscopes, white coats and an air of comforting authority whom we have admired and trusted from the first time they laid a cool hand on our feverish young foreheads? New tales of scandal, horror and wrong-doing by those people seem to break every day. And to think that we once thought them the nearest thing to saints on earth. We hear of the GP whose patients' bodies are being exhumed, we learn of the consultant gynaecologist who used his surgical knife with all the subtlety of a mowing machine inside women's bodies and left them broken and bleeding. And what could be more distressing than the Bristol case, in which the arrogance of two heart surgeons led to the deaths of tiny babies whose lives could have been saved if their parents had only known to take them somewhere else. (Boseley, 1998b)

The second article, under the caption '"Magic Bullet" trial to target brain cancer', provided a very positive review of how medical researchers and nuclear physicists were working on a project to offer 'new hope' to the thousands of people each year who are diagnosed with cerebral tumours (Radford, 1998). Assisted by the highly specialized paraphernalia of modern science (i.e. a nuclear accelerator), it is envisaged that 'boron neutron capture therapy' will be able to deliver a 'killer punch' to cancer cells.

Irving Zola (1972) has argued that the profession of medicine has displaced the influence of religion and the law in society. For Zola, medicine is now the pre-eminent instrument of social control. Many deviant behaviours have come under the gaze of the medical profession. The following series of hypothetical scenarios by Peter Conrad illustrates this point well:

> Consider the following situations: A woman rides a horse naked through the streets of Denver claiming to be Lady Godiva and after being apprehended by the authorities, is taken to a psychiatric hospital and declared to be suffering a mental illness. A well-known surgeon in a Southwestern city performs a psychosurgical operation on a young man who is prone to violent outbursts. An Atlanta attorney, inclined to drinking sprees, is treated at a hospital clinic for his disease, alcoholism. A child in California brought to a pediatric clinic because of his disruptive behavior in school is labelled hyperactive and is prescribed methylphenidate (Ritalin) for his disorder. A chronically overweight Chicago housewife receives a surgical intestinal bypass operation for her problem of obesity. Scientists at a New England medical center work on a million-dollar federal research grant to discover a heroin-blocking agent as a 'cure' for heroin addiction. What do these situations have in common? In all instances medical solutions are being sought for a variety of deviant behaviour or conditions ... the medicalization of deviance. (Conrad & Schneider, 1980, p28)

The medical profession has become the 'repository of truth' whereby the opinions of doctors hold great sway not only over anti-social behaviour, but also over the daily lives of the general population. Virtually all areas of our day-to-day activities, suggests Zola, have been infiltrated by medical representations of what is normal (health) and what is abnormal (ill-health). That is, our whole existence has become 'medicalized'.

The prevention of illness and the maintenance of health have become a pervasive standard by which many (if not all) behaviours (drinking, eating, work and leisure) are judged. This Crawford (1980) has described as 'healthism'. There has been an explosion of interest in exercise, jogging, diets, vitamins, health technology and anti-stress measures. There is an aggressive anti-smoking, anti-alcohol ethic, and a social stigma attached to perceptions of 'overeating'. There has also been a rise in the holistic health movement. These developments have resulted in the medicalization of the normal rather than just the deviant. The apparent promotion of 'autonomy' over one's life and health is in reality the promotion of oppression. Failure to maintain health is regarded as a failure of will. Healthy behaviour becomes the model for 'good living', and healthy people are 'good/ideal' citizens.

Psychiatric science

Medicalization has been rampant, especially in the area of human life that Szsaz (1972, 1973) calls 'problems with living'. Boyle (1993), argues that psychiatric medicine has perpetuated a 'scientific delusion' with respect to mental disorder. For Boyle, the psychosocial complexities that make up what we are as humans, the fallibility of psychiatric diagnosis and the fragility of bio-medical knowledge all combine to 'deconstruct' such so-called disease entities as schizophrenia.

However, Michael Stone, Professor of Clinical Psychiatry at the New York Columbia College of Physicians and Surgeons, comments that although psychiatry could still be considered to be immature and in need of incorporating humanistic precepts into its practice, it is still a progressive force in the alleviation of psychological distress. Stone (1998) suggests there have been three psychiatric revolutions initiated by psychiatrists. The first was the unchaining of the mad in the asylums, the second the development of psychoanalysis by Freud, and the third the application of pharmacology to psychological disorder. In the 1930s and 40s, new physical treatments (for example, psychosurgery and insulin therapy) were introduced, and then in the 1950s, the serendipitous 'discovery' of antipsychotic and antidepressant drug treatments reaffirmed the bio-medical base for the treatment of madness. There have been, Stone observes, more psychiatrists since 1955 than in all of the history of the discipline, and the discourse of psychiatric medicine has entered irreversibly into the culture of Western societies. That is, personal thoughts, behav-

iours, emotions and social values have been thoroughly 'psychia-
trized'.

The third revolution has been given a considerable boost by the
undeniably impressive progress made in medical diagnostic technology: computerized axial tomography, magnetic resonance imaging,
neuroimaging, photomicrography, positron emission tomography
and single photon emission tomography. Moreover, the third revolution has been further revitalized with a new wave of psychotropic
drugs such as the selective serotonin re-uptake inhibitors (SSRIs),
which were developed during the 1980s.

The most obvious and prolific example of the psychiatrization of
everyday life has been through the proliferation of the drug fluoxe-
tine hydrochloride (Prozac). Prozac, the first SSRI, is prescribed for
depression but has become, alongside the male impotency drug
Viagra, a principal 'lifestyle' remedy. In other words, just as Viagra
has been used to boost male sexual prowess (rather than merely to
address sexual dysfunction), so Prozac has become a 'mind-altering'
chemical used to combat the pressures and disappointments of ordinary human existence. Peter Kramer, an American professor of
psychiatry, champions Prozac as a 'personality improver'. In the
same way as Viagra is projected as providing men (and possibly
women) with extravagant orgasms, Kramer argues that taking
Prozac can make all of us feel 'better than well'. It is, for Kramer,
part of 'cosmetic psycho-pharmacology'. However, unlike somatic
cosmetic surgery, the SSRIs can be used not merely to restore but to
transform. Kramer highlights the transformative qualities of Prozac
with anecdotal depositions from his own practice. The following
extract refers to his patient 'Tess':

> Here was a patient whose usual method of functioning changed dramati-
> cally. She became socially capable, no longer a wallflower but a social
> butterfly. Where once she had focused on obligation to others, now she was
> vivacious and fun loving. Before she had pined after men, now she dated
> them, enjoyed them. (Kramer, 1993, p10–11)

Not only does scientific doctoring still prevail in the conscious-
ness of the public as the most significant 'world view', but in addition
the most irresolute area of medicine – psychiatry – is being seduced
by the lush trappings of the positivist paradigm. The individuation of

health is increased through new technologies and drugs as the physician's 'gaze' once again centres on the internal organs of the patient. That is, the social and political environment is displaced as the search for 'disease' concentrates on the infinitesimal within the human body.

Moreover, the third revolution has sanctified empiricism. In 1998, for example, an academic journal was inaugurated expressly with the aim of promoting 'evidence-based practice' in mental health. This journal (*Evidence-based Mental Health*) has the support of the Royal College of Psychiatrists, the British Psychological Society and the Royal College of Nursing. It is described as a 'sister' publication to the general medical journal *Evidence-based Medicine* and the nursing journal *Evidence-based Nursing*. The Editors of the journal proselytize on the merits of 'hard data' to support the practice of psychiatric medicine and clinical psychology:

> How much evidence is available on which to base mental health services? In fact, there is much evidence, which although difficult to find, is gradually being systematically reviewed by organisations such as the Cochrane Collaboration. Psychiatry was one of the first medical specialities to use extensively the randomised controlled trial, and one of the founding principles of the profession of clinical psychology in the 1950s was that practice should be based on the results of experimental comparisons of treatment methods. Multicentre randomised controlled trials showed the effectiveness of antidepressant and anitpsychotic drugs in the 1960s. The recognition of international variations in diagnostic practice led to the development of explicit diagnostic criteria such as the *Diagnostic and Statistical Manual*, third edition, of the American Psychiatric Association. (Geddes et al., 1997, p1483)

This evidence-based evangelism across the psychiatric disciplines of psychiatry, psychology and psychiatric nursing represents a rare open declaration of ideological compatibility and collaboration.

But the evidence-based movement in the psychiatric disciplines, which heralds the randomized controlled trial as the gold standard of research methodology and the purveyor of reliable 'truth', is based on a fundamentally flawed statistical formula. Robert Mathews (1998) divulges that 'tests of significance', the very heart of scientific analysis, are actually based on a subjective assessment of probability. That is, the setting of the dividing line of '0.05%' for evaluating the chance of an outcome being caused by an identified phenomenon was chosen in 1925 by Ronald Aylmer Fisher (who had attempted to correct a fault in a previous statistical theorem of Thomas Bayes) because it was 'convenient'. The consequence of this arbitrary calculation of what is and what is not significant is to exaggerate the importance of findings and produce false justifications for accepting highly implausible conclusions. This, argues Mathews, is why so many scientific and medical 'breakthroughs' discovered under experimental and/or laboratory conditions do not perform as such when in general circulation, and why there are so many contradictory results from studies examining the same problem.

Evolutionary theory is also giving sustenance to the positivist-empiricist renaissance in mental health, although this can be interpreted as moving the speciality 'beyond the medical model'. McGuire & Troisi (1998) go further by claiming that evolutionary theory is vying with the bio-medical model, which they describe as 'limited' and 'outdated'. Anthony Stevens and John Price (1996) argue that conventional psychiatry, as part of the medical kinship, has been led down the wrong epistemological path. They dispute the accepted psychiatric diagnostic classifications and treatments based on the notion of 'clinical entities'. Describing such 'conditions' as obsessive-compulsive disorder, depression and schizophrenia as 'illusions', they conjecture that symptoms displayed by those diagnosed as mentally disordered are in fact manifestations of adaptive strategies from early human development.

The production by medicine of lists of discrete diseases, caused by identifiable pathological changes in the body and susceptible to specific cures, was initiated by Hippocrates in the ancient world, and then refined by Thomas Sydenham in seventeenth-century England. By the end of the nineteenth century, Emil Kraepelin had assembled a comprehensive nosology of mental disorders. In the fourth version of the American Psychiatric Association's (1994) manual of mental disorders, there are 800 illness categories, ranging from 'Alzheimer's Disease' to 'Female Sexual Arousal Disorder'.

However, much of mental disorder, suggest Stevens & Price, results from adjustments to actual or projected loss of attachment or social rank. For example, what have become termed 'anxiety' and 'depression' are not disease entities but stem from the ways in which our ancestors had to deal with being marginalized from the group as a consequence of not being physically powerful or sexually enticing enough to succeed in mating. Losing rank meant a continual state of arousal in case of attack from either group members or external predators. Where an infant became 'detached' from its mother, survival was made more possible if it acted as despondent and inactive, conserving its physical resources, waiting to be reunited with a parent or adopted by a protective adult.

Using the work of Harpending & Sobus (1987), the evolutionary case is made for psychopathic behaviour by Stevens & Price. They accept that there is probably a genetic factor behind the creation of inveterate 'cheaters' and 'free-loaders' who have no conscience or sense of responsibility. However, they give weight to Harpending & Sobus's argument that the male psychopath will gain more mating partners than his prestige in society or his level of commitment warrants, by displaying engaging interpersonal qualities (such as humour). Equally, the relatively low-ranking female psychopath will attract extra attention from prospective mates and providers by appearing highly vulnerable and needy.

Schizophrenia, for Stevens & Price, has undeniable extra-evolutionary causative factors (genetic, biochemical and brain abnormalities). They argue, however, that schizophrenia (and this must, by inference, be the case for all of the psychiatric 'diseases' as well as presumably for all criminal behaviour) must be an adaptive mechanism. If it were not, they reason, natural selection would have removed schizophrenia from the human condition. Stevens & Price expound on their 'group-splitting hypothesis' to explain schizophrenia:

> A number of schizotypal characteristics, especially in their strong form as manifested in an acute schizophrenic episode, lend themselves to the charismatic leadership of a split-off and migrating group. These include the cognitive dissonance, the preoccupation with religious theme and belief in the occult, the disordered language and use of neologisms, the mood changes, the illusions and hallucinations which typify the condition. These peculiarities could well make it possible for a single individual to detach himself from the prevailing culture of his group to develop an entirely new, arbitrary belief system, which could be held with such conviction as readily to influence others when they are themselves in a disturbed or disaffected state. (Stevens & Price, 1996, p147)

So there we have it! Added to the teleological reductionism of the neo-Darwinian framework is charismatic functionalism. The qualities associated with charismatic leaders, which have enabled them throughout history to convince the 'disaffected' masses to follow them into the physical and/or social wilderness, have sprung from primeval circumstances whereby human groups divided because of growing numbers and intranecine conflict. That is, from the age of hunters and gatherers to the time of the Third Reich, a sizeable proportion of every distressed population will accompany the nearest deranged and incomprehensible madman or madwoman into uncharted territory.

As the science writer Kenan Malik (1998) notes, the objective and scientific status of evolutionary explanations may provide some interesting insights into human behaviour. Furthermore, although there remain major disagreements within evolutionary theorizing, the effect of the perspective overall has been to correct the simplistic and deterministic 'standard social science model' of regarding humans as being born with a 'blank slate'. Malik, however, argues that neo-Darwinian theory is based on a fallacy. He states that the 'mishmash of wild speculation, banal generalisations, circular arguments, giddy leaps of logic and uncorroborated assertions' (Malik, 1998, p8) not only undermine the rules of science that its adherents claim to follow, but also gain it nothing more than the standing of a 'New Age' religion.

Summary

Classical and positivist criminology, and the profession of medicine, have at root a conception of the 'flawed' individual in their analytical sights. For social contract theory (in both its old and new versions), humans have a propensity to shun their responsibilities and must be induced to accept these (with the promise of certain 'rights') or forced to conform by way of new 'community' legislation. Developments in science and evolutionary theory have refocused the gaze of the criminal justice system and the psychiatric disciplines back onto the innate qualities of the individual in the search for causative explanations of crime and madness.

There are, however, flaws in the theories. Not only are the precepts, logic and research underpinning these approaches to criminality and madness suspect, but also the scant regard given to the effect of social circumstances means that they cannot adequately explain variations in the incidence of crime and in the meanings attached to 'deviant' behaviour.

Chapter 5
Faulty societies

The second theoretical genre in the study of crime and deviancy has within it, as with the first, a number of distinct components, but here the focus of analysis moves away from the individual to that of society. That is, the various theories contained in this chapter concentrate on how either certain structures in society, society as a whole or the cultural norms of subgroups within society induce crime and deviance.

In a similar way to the identifying of 'faults' in the individual, the portrayal of society as imperfect leads to radical quests aimed at reducing crime. This time, however, rather than altering the constitution of the individual, it is society that requires modification, if not complete renewal. Moreover, the facts of crime are once again attributable to a knowable source and are considered amenable to (social) scientific manipulation.

Pathological structure

Social structure refers to the enduring configurations and divisions in society (for example, economic class, ethnicity, gender and age) and their associated role behaviours. Most criminals and mentally disordered people come from the same social pool. Put another way, similar social processes (for example, involving educational and material deprivation, prejudice and social exclusion) that are allied to criminality also seem to be associated with madness.

The effect of the social structure on health in general is incontrovertible. For example, the position in which an individual is situated within the social hierarchy based on class or wealth correlates with chronic disease and mortality. The further down the hierarchy a person is, the more disease-ridden he or she will be, and the earlier death will ensue. Apart from the important structural influences of gender, age and ethnicity on rates of mental 'ill-health', poorer people suffer from psychiatric problems far more than those who are successful (in terms of both financial and cultural capital) in society (Gomm, 1996). For example, there is a strong connection between (lower) social class and alcohol and drug addiction, schizophrenia, depression, Alzheimer's disease and personality disorder. A number of mental disorders occur more frequently amongst those further up the social scale, for example eating disorders, manic depression and the anxiety states (Cockerham, 1996).

It has, however, been argued that the higher incidence of schizophrenia and personality disorder amongst the lower stratum of society is a consequence of having these ailments rather than the result of particular social conditions (Robins, 1966; Britchenell, 1971). That is, 'social selection' is occurring as severely mentally disordered people either slide down into the poorer sections of society, or are not able to upgrade their social position, because of the disabling effects of their condition.

Sandra Bloom (1997) suggests that Western societies such as the USA are essentially 'sick' and that this sickness is exemplified in an addiction to violence. It is society rather than individuals that propagates violence. Although enacted by individuals, the aggressive act is a consequence of the values that a society generates. Values such as those associated with actual physical violence, or competitiveness in sport and at work, are inculcated into the individual via, for example, the educational system and the media.

When Nathaniel Lee, the seventeenth-century dramatist, was sent to Bethlem asylum, he protested against the right of the majority to make a judgement on his view of the world:

> They called me mad, and I called them mad, and damn them, they outvoted me. (quoted in Porter, 1987, p3)

The validity of this claim by the mad, that it is not they but everyone else who is crazy, is examined by Erich Fromm (1963). Fromm concludes that one form of society – capitalism – is indeed insane. Capitalism, for Fromm, has insuperable faults that indicate social pathology: the huge social and financial cost of conducting wars to protect markets; high levels of unemployment occurring regularly as a result of the vagaries of the economic system; the 'dumbing down' of human activities, and the displacement of face-to-face relationships because of mass entertainment; the propagation of a culture of materialism and commodity fetishism; and a loss of meaning to life.

From Fromm's perspective, homicide can be seen to be the outcome of specific flaws in the social and legal rules of a society. For example, the USA (and to some extent the same can be claimed of Australia and South Africa) is, because of its lax gun controls, more prey to multiple killings and a higher rate of suicide. Moreover, it is the brand of rampant capitalism that occurs in such countries as the USA that is ultimately responsible for encouraging the possession of guns. Excessive value is placed on individuality, ownership and an unregulated market (which allows large profits to be made on the manufacturing of weapons). Furthermore, the freedom to carry arms is sanctioned not only through the values of the capitalist system, but also in the constitution of the USA.

There are two basic types of social structure that sway rates of homicide. First, there are weaknesses in the 'control' structures of society that release people to carry out deviant acts. For example, the norms of a community may at times become 'disorganized', particularly if it is experiencing a high population turnover or significant level of material disadvantage. In such circumstances, the enforcement of law and order, and the replication of social norms, no longer apply consistently across the community.

Second, there are 'strains' in the structure of society that impel people to commit acts of deviance. For example, where people have become deprived of the accepted routes to social status and achievement (in terms of education and wealth), they may be forced to turn to crime in order to be 'successful'.

Messner & Rosenfeld (1999), in their review of the social-structural approach to homicide, conclude profoundly that the social production of homicide can be diminished if only a 'collective will' to do so is forthcoming. Reporting on the situation in the USA, they argue that the research to date on homicide demonstrates that:

> Persons with different sociodemographic characteristics exhibit distinctive
> levels of involvement in homicide as both victims and offenders. It also
> shows that variation in homicide rates can be accounted for, at least in part,
> by features of the social organisation of these collectivities. (Messner &
> Rosenfeld, 1999, p37)

For example, Messner & Rosenfeld claim that, in the USA, poverty is the major determinant of homicide for white people but not for black people. Residential segregation is the correlate for homicide amongst black people. They also refer to age and gender as structural factors that produce differential homicide patterns.

Conjecture in criminology about the conditions under which human performance is shaped by social structure has taken the path laid down by positivist theorists. Towards the end of the nineteenth century, and into the early part of the twentieth, the emerging discipline of sociology applied an 'organicist' model to the study of crime. Society was perceived as being analogous to the medical conception of the human body, which was regarded as being made up of interlocking and interdependent biological systems, as well as being in a state of perpetual and progressive change. Moreover, just as the profession of medicine had commenced its search for universal descriptions of 'normal' and 'abnormal' functioning in human physiology, and 'cause' and 'effect' relationships in corporeal malady, social scientists viewed society as either healthy or diseased. Whilst doctors treated dysfunctional organs to restore their patients to well-being, crime and other deviancies, such as prostitution, suicide, alcoholism, poverty and madness, represented social pathologies that had to be eradicated for the 'health' of the whole of society (Clinard & Meier, 1995).

The perspective of 'social pathology' not only used the rationalistic formulations of evolutionary biology and scientific medicine, but also incorporated a moralistic element. Those forces that undermined society's advancement were described as 'bad', and those which aided social progress were designated 'good' (Goode, 1996). 'Sickness' in society was evident at the level of the individual and social structure. Deviants were 'unhealthy' individuals who, as a consequence of faulty socialization, did not follow the norms, mores and laws of 'healthy' society. Certain social institutions were diseased because they were anachronistic or antagonistic to the steady but relentless improvements to the organization of society.

Social pathology theory lost its appeal on the basis that comparisons with human health and disease were fatuous and unsustainable; that is, societies do not behave in a fashion similar to that of organic material. Specifically, Clinard & Meier argue that:

[What] is pathological in a social sense is relative to norms, while what is pathological in the physiological sense is universal and unchanging. (Clinard and Meier, 1995, p103).

Clinard & Meier's notion of consistency in the medical understanding of physiology (and pathology) is somewhat questionable, but there can be little doubt that it is simplistic in the extreme to suggest that a virulent cancer in the human body is equivalent to increasing levels of violence in society. It is, however, interesting that contemporary medical rhetoric is imbued with social concepts – which are frequently related to violence. For example, medical practitioners talk of 'aggressive' therapies, whilst their patients refer to 'stabbing' pain.

Although the social pathologists had attempted to counteract theories that held individuals to be wholly at fault for their crimes or madness by giving prominence to the influence of society, the effect of this effort was limited. In practice, government policy was still focused on an imperfect social actor who was in need of 'moral' correction. However, a fundamental shift from concentrating on what was wrong with the individual (morally, biologically or psychologically) to an examination of the role of social structure as the deciding force of human conduct came about following the end of the First World War.

Social disorganization

The cataclysmic social and economic disorder, together with the horrifying personal experiences and privations of the 1914–18 'war to end all wars', had the long-term consequence of bringing into question a belief in universal values and a world order that had been established by the nations of Europe. The moral, social and political mandates of the Victorian age were to be irreparably damaged by the slaughter of millions of young people by nations projected as being civilized and at the forefront of social evolution. After 1918, the popular view became that this war had been based on spurious and illegitimate justifications, and propagated by incompetent and self-serving military and political leaders.

Moreover, during the period between the two World Wars, Western countries (particularly the USA, which had rapidly become a world power to rival and overtake the predominance of the British Empire) endured tremendous social change as a result of industrialization, urbanization and immigration. A further momentous influence on the social and economic assurances of nineteenth and early twentieth centuries was the 'Great Depression'. This began in the USA towards the end of the 1920s but spread rapidly to other industrialized countries. Share prices crashed, tens of thousands of businesses failed, there was a catastrophic decline in manufacturing output, both exports and internal consumption fell dramatically, and unemployment rose exponentially (Palmer, 1983).

In this climate, sociologists at the University of Chicago, over many decades, produced a sociological paradigm that attempted to come to terms with some of these social changes, especially those which seemed to be affecting (and affected by) the organization of life in the expanding and increasingly complex cities. Significantly, the 'Chicago School' was responsible for taking much further the argument that the role of society in the creation of criminal behaviour must be acknowledged:

> The Chicago School shifted its primary emphasis from individual pathology and individual problems of adjustment ... to seeing the social structure as the source of the problem. (Goode, 1996, p47)

It was, suggested these academics, the anarchic effects of unregulated civic planning, and massive demographic shifts from rural settings to living in sprawling industrial conurbations, that produced a high level of social disorganization. What they believed they observed in the cities was a problem of adjustment to change. An analogy was used with the ways in which biological organisms adjust to the imposition of either alien species or environmental modifications. Where intrusions occur over a prolonged period, the host organism can adjust. Where change is rapid, however, a whole genus may be irremediably damaged or even be wholly wiped out.

Countless species of animals, insects and birds have adapted successfully to alterations in climatic conditions when these have occurred over thousands of years (as with the various glacial epochs). Indeed, unless taking a 'creationist' position, this is the history of life on earth. However, when the temperature of the earth alters greatly and quickly (as is suggested by the 'meteorite' theorists about the sudden disappearance of the dinosaurs), some forms of life are caught out and either have to forfeit their previously favourable circumstances and exist in a hostile medium, or perish. In the same way as organisms can mutate and thereby survive when faced with evolutionary transformations, but cannot when the change is too fast or too imposing, so changes in the 'ecology' of human society can either be coped with or become destructive.

For social disorganization theorists such as Robert Faris and Warren Dunham (1965), the city can be broken down into a number of 'concentric zones' whose characteristics either enhance 'normality' or boost deviancy. In their model of the city, the zone at the geographical centre is the commercial sector, containing shops, offices, small factories and places of entertainment. Today, this area may also be occupied by the homeless, within whose ranks the mentally disordered will be disproportionately represented (Craig et al., 1995; Timms & Balazs, 1997). Those people without permanent residence take shelter in the nooks and crannies created by a bewildering display of architectural embellishment and anarchy typical of industrial and post-industrial design. Here, they ply their trade of begging or selling 'street papers' (such as *The Big Issue* in Britain).

The next zone identified by Faris & Dunham is typified by slum housing, ghettos and rented accommodation. In this area reside various groups of new immigrants, the lower working class (semi-skilled and unskilled workers, many of whom are only partially employed), and sections of the 'underclass' (the permanently unemployed, criminal recidivists, drug users and dealers, and prostitutes).

If and when the members of these groups are successful in terms of running businesses or finding employment, they have the opportunity to enter the third zone, which accommodates the 'stable working class' as well as former immigrants who are now more established within the social system.

In Britain, these last two zones have been to some extent 'gentri-fied'. That is, certain sections of the middle class (who are usually relatively young, either single or cohabiting, and without children) have 'converted' previously dilapidated housing into fashionable residences, thereby taking advantage of easy access to the centre of the city for work and entertainment.

Finally, situated on the edge of the city, there are the residential suburbs, the main habitation of the middle class. Today, however, there is also a growing minority of people who travel to the city from the countryside. Villages have seen the process of gentrification occur within their environs in the same way as it has occurred in the 'unfashionable' regions of the inner city.

Faris & Dunham argue that it was not the personalities and behaviour of the inhabitants that created the distinguishing features of these zones, but the other way round. That is, it was evident that the environment dictated how people behaved as each location maintained its specific identity despite the movement of groups (for example, Jewish immigrants being replaced by Hispanics in the USA, or Albanians succeeding North Africans in Europe) through its parameters. Moreover, even though high rates of mobility occur within the most unstable area (found principally in the second zone, but also in the first and third zones), a significant level of officially recorded crime and deviance continues. In fact, the pace of popula-tion movement causes the anonymity and social isolation that then produces the conditions under which crime and deviancy (including mental disorders such as schizophrenia) will flourish.

Interestingly, although criminal activity had grown to be a prob-lem in the 'core' areas of the modern city, electronic surveillance techniques have had the apparent effect of significantly reducing this, and arguably moved crime to regions on the outside of the busi-ness centre. Consequently, Faris & Dunham's observation from the 1960s that crime and deviancy are concentrated in areas around the centre of the city and become less so the further one travels away from the socially disorganized inner sections, remains appropriate in the twenty-first century.

It is also worth noting, however, that it is the perception of lawlessness in these highly mutable zones that appears to increase the fear of crime, rather than the issue merely being one of ecological instability. Taylor & Covington (1993) surveyed 1622 residents in 66 neighbourhoods of Baltimore City to assess fear levels. They reported that residents became alarmed at unexpected increases in the number of young people and ethnic minority groups. It was, argued Taylor & Covington, not the direct effects of the physical (dis)organization of the city that caused a rise in the level of fear, but a discerned upsurge in, for example, acts of incivility and unsupervised gatherings of adolescents.

Moreover, the social disorganization theorists have tended to focus on the crime and deviance of certain sections of the population – those who are situated at the bottom of the social hierarchy. That is, white-collar infringements (for example, fiddling expenses and tax evasion), which in the main do not register in the crime figures, are not taken into consideration. Hence, the premise that 'organized' social conditions encourage law-abiding and conformist behaviour may not be tenable. Furthermore, social disorganization theory can be portrayed as delivering a teleological argument. That is, the theory suggests that the lower end of the social spectrum embraces the majority of criminals and deviants because it exists in a state of social disorganization, but that it is socially disorganized because it contains many deviants and criminals (Traub & Little, 1994).

Surveys carried out in Britain have, however, confirmed a continued association between geographical location and mental disorder. For example, residents of cities or towns have a 50% greater chance of suffering from neuroses (especially anxiety and depression) and are twice as likely to experience psychotic disorder (particularly schizophrenia) than those who live in the countryside (Brindle, 1998).

Social strain

The idea that change leads to disorganization in society, which in turn produces criminal and deviant behaviour, is replicated in Robert Merton's work. Merton relied heavily on the precepts of Emile Durkheim (1858–1917), one of the founders of sociological thought and methodologies.

It was the sociology of Durkheim (1895/1964, 1897/1952) that was responsible for rectifying the reductionist view that construes human actions and social events as the consequence of individual volition. Football hooliganism, motivated school pupils, being in love, marriage, inner-city riots, feeling ill and even suicide (ostensibly the most personal of acts) were all seen to be a consequence of social factors. Durkheim regarded the structures, roles and institutions of a society as all operating cohesively and functionally for that society. When conflict occurs in society (for example, between employers and trade unions, feminists and patriarchs, rich and poor, or blacks and whites), compromise and adaptation will eventually take place at a slow and orderly pace, and social stability will therefore be maintained. In this way, social evolution is analogous to the Darwinian approach to human development.

Social order is further maintained through the process of socialization, which reproduces common values and beliefs amongst most of the population and from one generation to another. Morality, for Durkheim, is maintained through the operation of a 'collective conscience'. The collective conscience, an abstract but nevertheless potent phenomenon, confers the moral standpoint of a society and puts pressure on individuals to conform to its norms. Here, Durkheim is invoking the notion that society itself is greater than the 'sum of its parts' and that individuals are social products.

The conceptualization of society as having an existence beyond the aggregate of the behaviours and thoughts of its citizens, and of individuals as being the consummation of social forces, raises questions concerning the singularity of the 'self':

> In every human group, the boundaries of an individual's sense of 'self' are not necessarily the same as the boundaries of their body – and their sense of personal identity extends far beyond the borders of their skin ... Other 'symbolic skins' that help to define a person's sense of 'self' may include their cars, the outer limits of their suburbs and cities, the membership of their ethnic group, or even the borders of their nation state. (Helman, 1994, pp16–17)

According to Durkheim, those who object to the dominant ideology of a society are looked upon as deviants. The 'collective sense of self' means that they are not merely transgressing some distant and disconnected rule, but also undermining the community of which they are an integral part.

Paradoxically, however, deviancy may for Durkheim have a useful purpose in society. That is, a moral appreciation of what is 'good' in society depends on the opposite being available for scrutiny. The argument is that by recognizing and categorizing socially disruptive behaviours, the norms of society are reaffirmed. For example, the apparent drunken and violent conduct displayed by English football supporters in Marseilles during the 1998 World Cup was transmitted by the attending media throughout dozens of countries with newspaper headlines such as 'England fans rampage' (Duncan, 1998). The subsequent furore amongst politicians and the 'law-abiding public' served to underscore what was and was not acceptable within the 'national character' of this particular country.

Merton (1938) applied Durkheim's concept of 'anomie' to the issue of antisocial behaviour. Anomie is the state of 'normlessness' that an individual may experience when confronted by profound and rapid transformation in the way in which society is organized, and in the belief systems and moral guidelines it propagates. In situations in which the orderly administration and integration of social institutions is irresolute, the consequential social disorder may cause (some) people to experience debilitating feelings of aimlessness, insecurity and despair. Anomie may also lead to suicide.

For Merton, there is, however, a particular problem when the norms and expectations of the individual do not correspond with the reality of his or her social existence. For example, in the West, material wealth and occupational advancement are given high value, and their achievement is portrayed as the inevitable outcome of the effort of the individual. But, if despite application and diligence, an individual does not reach these goals, illegitimate strategies may be used. That is, if the means to fulfil the values of 'normal' society (economic success and promotion) are severely hampered by social disadvantage (for example, inequalities in schooling, racism, sexism and ageism), 'strain' occurs in both the individual and society.

According to Merton (1938), people react to this strain in a number of ways:

1. Conformity. There is an acceptance of both the values and means of achieving these values, notwithstanding the fact that

most will fail in their endeavours as there is only limited 'room at the top'. The majority of the population follow this route.

2. Ritualization. Here people acquiesce to the means of achieving 'success', as determined by social norms, but do so without an end game in sight in terms of achievement – for example, the employee who 'plods' through his or her working life.

3. Retreatism. Both values and means of achieving what is regarded highly in society are relinquished in favour of an alternative lifestyle – for example, 'new-age travellers' and employees who opt for demotion in order to concentrate on their social and personal interests.

4. Rebellion. A critical view of the social system is taken, and its means and values are rejected, but instead of 'retreating', attempts are made to introduce radical amendments to its structure and ideology. For example, social campaigners may set up their own political party to gain power and thereby change society, or alternatively they may instigate a revolution.

5. Innovation. The attainment of socially decreed outcomes such as wealth is accepted, but the means used are not within the moral or legal framework of society's norms. Deviants and criminals are therefore innovators.

The important point to acknowledge with Merton's analysis of the causes of deviancy and criminality is that it is the 'normal' values of society and the common practices of social institutions that are responsible (Goode, 1996). The corollary of this approach, therefore, is that rather than focusing on, and altering the behaviour of, the deviant, adjustments (perhaps dramatic ones) have to be made to the organization and ideology of mainstream society.

However, Giddens advises circumspection with regard to the assumption that there is unanimity between those at the top of the society's hierarchy and those further down the social ladder over achievement:

We should be cautious about the idea that people in poorer communities aspire to the same level of success as more affluent people. Most tend to adjust their aspirations to what they see as the reality of their situation. (Giddens, 1997, p178)

Giddens warns also of assuming that discordance between aspiration and the opportunity to achieve what is aspired to occurs only among the underprivileged. He points out that criminal activity thrives amongst the wealthy, although this may take a form different from that of the less privileged classes.

Subcultures

The link between disorganized and/or strained urban areas and crime has been made by a number of other deviancy theorists. Albert Cohen (1955), for example, attempted to understand why inner-city areas seemed to spawn delinquent subcultures. In particular, Cohen explored the frustration, later to be identified by Merton, experienced by people whose access to the means of achieving social success is denied. Cohen believed that belonging to groups that propagated and valued patterns of behaviour alternative to those perceived by society at large as being acceptable allowed disadvantaged young people to gain high status and respectability.

David Matza (1964, 1969) developed the concept of 'delinquent drift' as an explanation of how deviants can commit infringements against the norms and expectations of society without the 'strain' of feeling guilt and shame. For Matza, delinquents counteract the controlling effect of legal, moral and social rules by a process of reclassification. Crimes can, therefore, be committed with impunity because individual rule-breakers have determined that particular laws or conventions are irrelevant to their social situation. This subjective expunging of the codes and laws of society produces the precondition for the individual deviant to 'drift' into a subculture of delinquency.

There is, however, a major problem with causative explanations that rely on notions of 'strain' and 'disorganization':

> how was it that not all lower class youth embraced the delinquent subculture
> nor chose the same kind of deviant solution despite being subjected to simi-
> lar strains of social disorganisation? (Walklate, 1998, p23)

Indeed, this question of 'Why do some people commit crimes but others do not even though it would seem that all are exposed to similar socio-environmental influences?' pervades every explanatory framework in criminology.

The contribution of Richard Cloward and Lloyd Ohlin (1960) offered one way of coming to terms with this conundrum. They observed that delinquency was dependent upon not only the existence of the socially sanctioned means to achieve success, but also the degree to which illegitimate practices were accessible. That is, in some circumstances, individuals may be thwarted in their endeavours to be respected by the established purveyors of social accreditation (for example, educationalists and employers), but they may not have the chance or the practical resources to engage in a level of criminal activity that would bring sufficient reward (either social or pecuniary). Moreover, the very personal attributes (for example, imagination and initiative) that may lead to *de jure* social prosperity are, arguably, also necessary for an auspicious criminal career (Allsop, 1961).

For those caught without any means to succeed in society, impetuosity and self-destructiveness may be the only choice:

> some poor and highly transient neighbourhoods may lack any form of opportunity – legal or otherwise. Here delinquency often surfaces in the form of *conflict subcultures* where violence is ignited by frustration and a desire for fame and respect. Alternatively, those who fail to achieve success, even by criminal means, may sink into *retreatist subcultures*, dropping out through abuse of alcohol and other drugs. (Macionis & Plummer, 1997, p211, original emphases)

Homeless mentally disordered people may bcome contaminated by these conflict and retreatist subcultures, whose members are either actively antagonistic towards the dominant culture or withdraw from it to form their own (deviant) norms and values. For mad people, the only available social position in these circumstances is the lowest stratum within the alcoholic, drugged, violent and vagrant population of the inner-city areas.

Conflict and power

A vital constituent in the process of creating and maintaining the structure of a society is power. Although there are many theories that use power and conflict as their focus of analysis, the work of Karl Marx (1818–1883) has provided a significant explanatory framework with which to examine how powerful groups maintain their dominant positions in the social hierarchy.

For Marxist theorists, power is expropriated by the section of society that owns the resources of production. In capitalist societies, the bourgeoisie (i.e. the dominant class) have gained ownership of industry and commerce. The powerful interests of this class permeate all social and political organizations and influence what is considered to be important in human relationships. That is, the ideology of capitalism infiltrates all aspects of an individual's social and personal life.

Marxism was to debunk the notion that the law, and social rules in general, reflect a common ('consensual') agreement across society about what are acceptable and what are unacceptable 'norms'. For Marxists, there cannot be a set of behaviours that reflect the interests and views of most of the population as, no matter what form society takes (unless it is communist), conflict exists between the various layers of the social structure. In capitalist societies, it is the bourgeoisie who are in discord with the proletariat (the working class).

The desires of the mass of the population (for example, to have washing machines, new cars, exotic holidays and even 'good health') are, far from being under the free will of the individual, fashioned by the capitalist class. We accept as 'normal' the work ethic, paid labour, material possession and the legitimacy of the social hierarchy – all of which are necessary for the survival of the capitalist system:

> To ensure a skilled and willing labour force, labourers [i.e. workers] need to be trained to acquire skills but they also need to be willing to accept their subordinate position in society. (Layder, 1994, p40)

Moreover, as Lukes (1974) has observed, not only does the social system dictate what is on the menu of life, but also what we believe should be on that menu in the first place is also fabricated for us.

In the main, structuralist theory regards the state (government and political organizations and legal, health and educational institutions) as a conduit for the interests of the dominant class. Agencies of the state, such as the institutions of law and order, are seen to impose definitions of normality and deviance. Conflict, is, for the Marxist, managed in the interests of the powerful through the operations of the state and its agencies. That is, central and local government, the judiciary and the police, as well as the media and educational and medical institutions, provide the means (practical and ideological) whereby conformist behaviour is encouraged and actions that threaten capitalism are regulated.

For conflict theorists, it is those who obstruct capitalist production or attack its values (that is, private ownership, the work ethic, individual effort, materialism, ascribed authority and rationalism) who are labelled as deviant (Spitzer, 1980). In particular, those who damage or steal property are singled out for special attention by the agencies of social control and punishment. The cause of crime is, for these theorists, not the 'fault' of the individual or the consequence of partaking in subcultural activities, but the harsh and abusive nature of capitalism. Erich Goode summarizes the Marxist analysis of the root of high crime in industrialized societies:

> Capitalism is a ruthless, and exploitative system. At its foundation is an economy that depends on a high rate of unemployment, which in turn means that many poor, out-of-work people have no alternative but to commit crime to survive ... Even the general cultural climate is based on ruthlessness, promoting a culture of crime and violence, thereby inducing extraordinary high rates of rape, murder, assault, and robbery. Moreover, the Marxist would say, the fact that capitalism generates a large, poor, powerless underclass whose members lack many basic human amenities, makes it necessary for them to engage in criminal behavior for their sheer survival. (Goode, 1996, p165)

If this form of conflict theory is adopted, then, to a large extent, what criminals do and how society should react to their actions is unimportant when formulating social policy. Although not even the most ardent Marxist theorist would be able to sustain the argument that it is possible to make crime extinct, criminal behaviour could be substantially reduced by removing the inequalities in society. To do this, however, social revolution would be necessary in order to remove the mode of production (that is, capitalism) that is generating inequality, and replace it with an equitable economic and social system. So far, the creation of such a society has proven rather illusive.

It is somewhat ironic that Marx himself did not regard crime as an example of (working) class insurrection against the ruling class (Croall, 1998). For Marx, criminals were members of an unproductive underclass – the lumpenproletariat. This group were parasitic on both the working and the capitalist classes, hardly an empathic view of criminality or one consistent with the 'vulgar' Marxist assumption that deviants are proto-revolutionaries. Frederick Engels (1820–1895), Marx's long-term co-revolutionary theorist, did, however, acknowledge a more direct relationship between social inequalities and crime. At a time when England was rapidly industrializing, Engels used his own observations and official government statistics to connect the 'condition of the working class' to a rising crime rate, most of which arose within the proletariat itself:

> the social order makes family life almost impossible for the worker. In a comfortless, filthy house, hardly good enough for mere night shelter, ill-furnished, often neither rain-tight nor warm, a foul atmosphere filling rooms over-crowded with human beings, no domestic comfort is possible ... And children growing up in this savage way, amidst these demoralizing influences, are expected to turn out goody-goody and moral in the end! Verily the requirements are naive, which the self-satisfied bourgeois makes upon the working man! The contempt for the existing social order is most conspicuous in its extreme form – that of offences against the law ... Hence with the extension of the proletariat, crime has increased in England, and the British nation has become the most criminal in the world. (Engels, 1845/1969, pp158–9)

Theories with 'conflict' at the heart of their understanding of how society is structured, although not indulging in the biological or psychological reductionism of early positivistic criminology, maintain a conceptualization of the criminal as 'pathological'. In this instance, however, the deviance is socially contrived rather than being the outcome of the individual's constitution:

> the stress remains on the way in which men's criminal behaviour and behaviour in general are *determined*. It may be that the criminal behaviour, for example, of thieves, is determined by the unequal possession and distribution of wealth in a society; or it may be that the political deviance of contemporary radicals (prepared to face the force of law) is determined by the monopoly of defining power by the state or the rule-enforcers. But the overwhelming impression is one of determination at the expense of *purpose* and *integrity* ... conflict theorists see a relatively simple relationship between power and interest, and the consciousness of men ... such a conception undermines or understresses an alternative view of men as purposeful creators and innovators of action. (Taylor et al., 1981, p 267, original emphases)

Specifically, argue Taylor et al., the conflict theorists make the mistake of viewing crime as being directly the outcome of inequalities in society and the abuse of power, rather than being the result of individual volition in response to these inequalities. That is, for these authors, a well-developed theory of criminology must incorporate both social structure and human motivation.

Moreover, the concept of 'the state' in Marxist theory has been greatly criticised (Sumner 1997). There is frequently, for example, an incongruous conflation of the term as first an abstraction, second a varying number of organizations, and third a conscious, thinking and acting organism. Furthermore, as Nicos Poulantzas (1978) has pointed out, far from the state and the bourgeoisie being mutually supportive, the interests of the state and the interests of people with economic power may at times appear antithetical. For example, a government may institute laws that ensure a basic wage for employees, against the wishes of employers. However, the social system itself is not being dismantled in these circumstances as the essential values and practices of capitalism remain intact. Moreover, although professionals such as psychiatrists may not be aligned unequivocally with the dominant class, they (and their nursing co-collaborators) either directly or indirectly shore up the capitalist system through their association with the functions of the state.

Theories that analyse the use and abuse of power in society are, however, not restricted to Marxism. Feminism – in all its variations – has in particular contributed to an understanding of the organization of power beyond that of social class, especially that which is associated with patriarchy (Smart, 1976). The most conspicuous, but until relatively recently virtually completely ignored, of all observations to make from the raw statistical data on crime is that most of it is committed by men. Moreover, the discovery of 'new' types of crime give further evidence of men's oppression of women. These include rape in marriage, stalking, domestic violence and sexual abuse in childhood.

Furthermore, the commonly assumed leniency of the courts towards female offenders may be a myth. Although the evidence is somewhat sketchy and inconsistent, it is argued that women who appear before the courts, which by and large replicate the prejudices and inequalities of a male-dominated society, are considered to be flagrantly and reprehensibly deviant. This is because they have not only broken the law, but also failed to adhere to their 'appropriate' gender role (Gelsthorpe, 1997). Therefore, a woman may be actually treated worse by the courts than may a man, even though both have committed the same misdemeanour. However, as with Taylor et al.'s criticism of Marxist theory, this is, by blaming patriarchy for the 'maleness' of crime and construing women as victims of men and their criminality, socially deterministic and does not give enough credence to human volition. For example, the questions of how much individual women may contribute to their 'victim' status, and how many men are innocent of any degree of oppression (or are indeed possibly victims themselves of the injustices of either, for example, female cruelty or biased courts in divorce settlements) cannot be easily accounted for within the patriarchy thesis.

Cybersociety

The third millennium arguably brings with it far greater disorganization, strain and restructuring than that experienced even in the twentieth century (or indeed in any foregoing epoch):

> With the development of mass communication, particularly electronic communication, the interpenetration of self-development and social systems, up to and including global systems, becomes ever more pronounced. The 'world' in which we now live is in some profound respects thus quite distinct from that inhabited by human beings in previous periods of history. (Giddens, 1991, p5)

Transnational computer networks have the potential to reconfigure the fabric of all societies. This projected new form of community, created by computer-mediated communication (that is, the Internet), Steven Jones (1995) terms 'cybersociety'. The state in any particular country will have less and less sway over the values, norms and behaviours of its citizens in the electronically driven 'global village'. On the other hand, globalization may merely replicate the structures (and inequalities) of the nation state but on a bigger scale.

In cybersociety, an individual's ontological identity (what he or she believes to be the essence of his or her 'self') will, far from being relatively 'fixed' and knowable, constantly mutate. The electronification of interpersonal communication is altering how people see themselves and how they relate to each other. In cybersociety, there are few if any restrictions or guidelines on the presentation of one's 'self' to the outside world.

As a disembodied and deregulated entity, we can literally be who we want to be at any point in time. The usual non-verbal and environmental clues and feedback, which help to substantiate what we are as humans and contextualize intended meanings, are replaced by the social void of cyberspace. Where video cameras are used to supplement cyber-communication with visual images, there is still an esoteric code of interpersonal behaviour that needs to be learned, and which does not fully compensate for the absence of the interlocutor's physical presence.

The Internet has also spawned novel configurations of criminality and deviancy. Fraudulent financial dealings, illegal trading in weapons, drug trafficking and the distribution of pornography, for example, become easier to carry out electronically and can operate globally. Criminal and deviant groups, such as drug addicts, child abusers and neo-Nazis, can also have a greater degree of freedom to contact each other, deliver their propaganda and recruit more participants.

The antisocial nature of these activities may be neutralized by their easy accessibility and existence in a public arena. Most 'terrestrial' crime and deviancy is, by its very nature, hidden from view. Those who do indulge in crime and deviancy behaviour tend to do so furtively. Transgressing social convention in cyberspace (if only to the point of gaining information) is as easy as switching on a computer.

What are the mental health problems for members of cybersociety? A two-year study of the social and psychological effects of the Internet by researchers at Mellon University in Pittsburgh found that, from a sample of 169, greater usage resulted in higher levels of depression and loneliness (Kraut et al., 1998). Case study research into the addictive effects of technology by Mark Griffiths (1999) suggests that persistent use of the Internet produces a psychological 'high', and when use is curtailed, withdrawal symptoms can occur as a result of chemical changes in the body. A significant minority of users may become addicted to the Internet in the same way as other addicts do with drink, tobacco, drugs or gambling. Griffiths observes that, just as occurs with these other forms of addiction, computer junkies could have serious problems in their personal lives because of their obsession.

Philip Zimbardo, Professor of Psychology at Stanford University and founder of the Stanford Shyness Clinic, comments that what he describes as the 'silent prison' of reticent behaviour is being generated by the spread of electronic communication (in Mihill, 1997). For Zimbardo, electronically induced shyness had reached epidemic proportions by the late 1990s. Computers, he argues, may in the future erode the 'social glue' of casual conversation. Zimbardo suggests that, alongside a rise in impersonal contact in the business sphere (for example, using 'cash machines' instead of conversing with a bank clerk), the increasing use of e-mail, mobile telephones, lap-top computers and computer games is significantly reducing 'real' interchanges between friends, relatives and colleagues. He argues that it may eventually be possible to function in our work and personal lives without ever talking directly to anyone.

For Zimbardo, however, shyness may not only lead to the sufferer losing out in the job market but also in his or her personal relationships. Using data from his own research into a group of ten murderers (Zimbardo & Bertholf, 1977), eight of whom were classified as shy, he suggests that social reserve (which he predicts will increase dramatically in the world of electronic 'virtuality') is associated with outbursts of uncontrolled violence.

Summary

The 'faulty society' explanatory genre is, as with those perspectives attempting to discover faults in the individual, ultimately deterministic and singular in its search for the causation of crime and madness. This time, however, instead of genes, biochemicals and personality traits, specific elements in the way in which society is managed and arranged, or a particular mode of production (especially capitalism), are used to explain transgressions from the norm.

The way in which society is structured, and the circumstances in which people live, undoubtedly play a part in the production of crime and madness. The globalization and electronification of commerce and communication is yielding further influences on human conduct. Cybersociety will act as a catalyst for an expansion in organized crime and offer a venue for the promulgation of deviant lifestyles.

Chapter 6
Faulty images

Perspectives that can loosely be placed under the rubric of constructionism (or 'constructivism') are evaluated in this chapter, and make
up the third explanatory genre for the subject of crime and deviancy.
Specifically, these perspectives are labelling theory, moral panic
theory and postmodernist conjecture.

Constructionism has not only been of major importance to
the comprehension of criminality and deviance, but also impregnated much of the professional and academic theorizing concerning mental disorder. This permeation of constructionism into
criminology and the mental health industry is paradoxical,
however, as the core tenets of this genre are epistemologically and
politically in opposition to the other science-dependent frameworks discussed earlier. What this third field of thought does have
in common with the other genres is that it also lays the blame for
criminality and deviancy at a number of specific targets – this time
the powerful in society and their acolytes, including the psychiatric disciplines.

There are a number of further ambiguities that can be observed
in how the genre is applied to mental disorder. For example,
elements of the constructionist genre are used not only by critics
external to the mental health industry, but also by internal dissidents
from that field, to point out how the psychiatric disciplines erect
'false imagery'. However, as is elaborated further in Chapter 8, the
psychiatric establishment has also used constructionism, conspicu-
ously in its attack on what it has portrayed as the defamatory and
injudicious role of the media in fabricating public fear about the
mentally disordered.

Labelling

The major antipositivistic influence on the understanding of criminal behaviour was advanced by the symbolic interactionists of the Chicago school. This variety of sociological thought, inaugurated by George Herbert Mead (1863–1931), focused on interpreting the impact of society on certain conducts by examining the significance (or 'symbolism') of human interaction. For Mead, language separated human society from all other forms of animal collective life. Communication between humans is fundamentally different from the transmission of messages through 'gesturing' as happens in the animal world. Human communication has 'meaning', and the participants have the potential to 'understand' what is being transmitted, by placing themselves in the position of those with whom they are communicating.

Moreover, through a process of interactive reflexivity, humans reformulate the meanings given to aspects of their social and physical environment. That is, the sense we make of our lives involves an active and reciprocal process of communication whereby each participant: sends messages to which he or she has attached particular meanings; has those messages interpreted by the other person(s); receives back modified versions of these messages; and in turn adjusts, in one way or another, the 'sense' that he or she now makes of these messages – and so on.

If humans are to be depicted, as they are by the symbolic interactionists, as conscious, thoughtful, intentional and able to interpret their personal, social and physical surroundings 'meaningfully' (and thereby influence their environment), then research techniques different from those of positivism are required. These are, principally, participant observation, in-depth interviewing and the analysis of 'discourse'. All of these methods are designed to 'interpret' the subjective significance that humans give to their social world rather than establish objective causal relationships between pre-given phenomena.

For Mead, the 'self', configured by language, is the locus of psychosocial activity. It is at this level that the interplay of individual mental computations, reflexive interactions with others, and social forces occurs. That is, the 'self' is the vital repository for an ongoing dialogue between internal mechanisms (psychological) and external (interpersonal and social) influences. This dialogue is represented by an inner conversation between two interactive elements of the 'self' – the 'I' and the 'me':

> The 'I' is the thinking and acting subject, the creator and initiator, literally the ego. The 'me' is the objective self, the self upon which the 'I' reflects, it is the self thought of in other situations and in other times and places, both real and imagined. Most importantly it is the aspect of self which is an expression of the gaze of others upon it ... So society flows into the individual via the 'me' and is simultaneously constructed and re-constructed by the 'I'.
> (Waters, 1994, p25)

Therefore, symbolic interactionists perceive humans as both creating and being created by society. Moreover, the fully developed 'self', in which the 'I' and the 'me' have successfully integrated, is also in harmony with society. A successfully integrated self is one that has been able to empathize with the roles and expectations of the social groups to which he or she belongs, and to society overall. That is, 'I–me' union moves the social actor from selfishness to the internalization and understanding of the 'generalized other'. Therefore, the mature 'self' both reflects, and is a reflection, of society.

Symbolic interaction gave rise to the 'labelling' (or 'social reaction') theory of Edwin Lemert (1951) and Howard Becker (1963), which portrays 'crime' not in terms of inherent characteristics (biological or psychological), but as sets of actions or beliefs that attract the tag of 'deviancy' because of how 'moral entrepreneurs' (Becker, 1974) react when these behaviours are observed. Labelling theory took from symbolic interactionism the notion that both the meaning given by the individual to his or her behaviour, and the reactions of others, combine to define that behaviour. However, what was paramount for the labelling theorists was that where those observing the behaviour were powerful (particularly if representing such agencies of social control as the police and psychiatry), their interpretation would displace that intended by the individual.

What the labelling theorists argue is that an action is not in itself either 'normal' or 'deviant' until meaning has been ascribed to it by observers of the act in question. Thus, car theft, burglary or even murder are not innately 'bad' unless given the value of 'badness' by others. Behaviours that attract the description of 'madness' are not intrinsically threatening to the social order unless construed as such by others. Moreover, a massive amount of rule-breaking can occur in society, but unless this is observed (or 'reacted to'), it does not count as deviancy. Consequently, the process of labelling can be regarded as manufacturing categories of deviance and/or overstating the menace of certain behaviours or conditions to society.

By the 1960s, the labelling approach to deviancy was triumphant over the prevailing belief that those who transgressed social norms were in some way different from the rest of the population, either because of inborn characteristics or because of structural disadvantage. The heritage of Mead's interactionism, with its emphasis on the 'self' as the crucial point of study in order to understand human behaviour and social processes, meant that deviance could be considered to be a negotiated outcome of human interaction as opposed to a 'fact'. This, therefore, leads to a relativist position whereby what is deviant for one person (or group) may not be so for others, and that contexts, time and the identity of the 'labeller' are elementary factors in the construction of deviant categories and careers:

> different groups judge different things to be deviant. This should alert us to the possibility that the person making the judgement of deviance, the process by which that judgement is arrived at, and the situation in which it is made may all be intimately involved in the phenomenon of deviance. (Becker, 1963, p3)

The distinction is made by Lemert (1967) between primary and secondary stages in the 'career' of the deviant. Over a period of time, an individual is socialized into a permanent deviant identity. Primary deviance occurs in a wide variety of situations and, according to Lemert, is limited in its effect on the human psyche. That is, the common rule-breaking indulged in by perhaps a majority of the population at one time or another (breaking the speed limit whilst driving our cars, using equipment or services belonging to our employer without permission, taking 'soft' drugs) has only a negligible effect on how we perceive ourselves or are viewed by others. This is especially the case if our deviant actions go unnoticed by other people. But if our actions are uncovered, and if the reaction of others and the processes we go through as a consequence of being 'found out' are disapproving, isolating, long-lasting and stigmatizing, our 'deviant career' (Goffman, 1963) has begun.

Moreover, the inauguration of a deviant career may be signified by what Harold Garfinkel (1968) describes as a 'degradation ceremony' (for example, the removal of all personal possessions on entry to prison, or being made to wear hospital clothes on admission to a psychiatric hospital). It is at this 'secondary' stage that the label starts to define the person, separating him or her from 'normal' society. Furthermore, the clustering of people with similar labels in such 'total institutions' (Goffman, 1961) as gaols and asylums will create a self-perpetuating process of socialization whereby the deviant identity is reinforced. Social control in these circumstance can be seen as the source of deviancy rather than a consequence of it (Lemert, 1967).

In this sense, the labelling that occurs at the secondary stage is so influential on the 'self', and on future behaviour, that the original causes of the deviant act become irrelevant. That is, labelling theory does not provide a causal explanation for crime. The reasons for someone becoming a criminal, a homosexual, a drug addict, or mad in the first place, are seen to be of only perfunctory interest to those studying social reaction.

Becker himself acknowledges the limitations of the perspective:

> The original proponents of the [labelling] position ... did not propose a solution to the aetiological question. They had more modest aims. They wanted to enlarge the area taken into consideration in the study of the deviant phenomena by including in it activities of others than the allegedly deviant actor. (Becker, 1974, p42)

What is also occurring in the process of secondary labelling, observes Paul Rock (1997), is the 'symbolic synthesis' of the myths, prejudices, professional values and assumptions of the agents of social control with which the deviant comes into contact (police officers, judges, medical practitioners and prison officers). The deviant is then obliged to fashion his or her behaviour around the symbols used by those who are sitting in judgement. Deviants become what those judging them expect them to be.

With respect to mental disorder, it was the application of labelling theory by Thomas Scheff (1966) that has been the most fascinating. What Scheff proposed was that mental disorder was merely 'residual' rule-breaking. That is, when all other categories of deviance have been exhausted, the label of 'madness' will be put to use. This was particularly the case when the presentation of an 'unacceptable' behaviour was persistent and had not attracted an alternative deviancy tag. For Scheff, the remnant and lowly connotation of the label 'mad' was likely to stick permanently to the individual. As a result, the mentally disordered person had little choice but to accept the proffered stereotype and act accordingly. In Erving Goffman's (1963) terms, the individual who is stigmatized by a label such as mental disorder becomes socially discredited and discreditable, and has his or her identity 'spoiled' by the attitude of the 'normals'.

Stigma is explained (teleologically) by Goffman as any condition or attribute that draws towards it social condemnation and sanctions of one sort or another. Goffman describes three different types of stigma, the first of which are 'abominations of the body' (a visible naevus or physical deformity). Second come 'blemishes of individual character' (alcoholism, criminality, homosexuality, unemployment and mental disorder). Third, there is 'tribal stigma', whereby a group will be outcast on the basis of race, nationhood or religion.

Lindsay Prior (1993) notes that Scheff's analysis has, over a long period of time, been incorporated into the professional training syllabuses of both psychiatric social work and mental health nursing. However, it is not just social workers and nurses who call upon the theories of labelling. For example, Kay Redfield Jamison, a psychologist and Professor of psychiatry at John Hopkins School of Medicine, Baltimore, and herself a sufferer of manic depression, comments on the endemic stigmatization of mentally disordered people:

> It would be hard to overstate the degree of stigmatisation faced by those who have mental illness: it is pervasive in society, rampant in the media, and common within the medical profession. Psychiatric illnesses, although widely prevalent and usually amenable to treatment, too often are minimized or misconceived. Virtually every patient who has been diagnosed with severe depression, manic depression, or schizophrenia will, given a sympathetic forum, relate numerous hurtful comments or actions based solely on carrying a psychiatric diagnosis. (Jamison, 1998, p1053)

Roland Littlewood (1998), consultant psychiatrist and Professor of anthropology and psychiatry at University College, London, records that there is some evidence that a popular (mis)understanding of, and reaction to, mental disorder can impair the potency of medical treatment. The findings of comparative studies of cultures in which there is less stigma of mental disorder with those which have a high rate of intolerance indicate that, in the latter, the prognosis for sufferers may be worse. Littlewood, however, admits that such studies are rare and conceptually problematic given the controversy surrounding the universality or relativity of psychiatric diagnostic categories.

The infiltration of perspectives from the constructionist camp into psychiatric orthodoxy is no better exemplified than by a policy initiative from the World Psychiatric Association (WPA) aimed at fighting head on the stigma and discrimination associated with schizophrenia. In his account of the initiative, Norman Sartorius (1998), consultant psychiatrist and President of the WPA, declares that stigma and discrimination are the greatest obstacles to the successful rehabilitation of people with severe mental disorder and to their enjoyment of an acceptable quality of life. Moreover, he suggests that psychiatrists have a responsibility to examine their own prejudices towards such illnesses as schizophrenia and must become more aware of how stigma affects their patients and families. Furthermore, he recommends that psychiatrists should engage actively in political action, dealing vigorously with any signs of prejudice in the public domain. Sartorius also argues for the 'important topic' of stigma to enter prominently and enduringly into the discourse of the psychiatric disciplines.

This wide usage of social reaction theory within the mental health field occurs despite the fundamental criticisms that, as a model, it contains little understanding of, or explanation for, the initial rule-breaking behaviour. Indeed, social reaction theory can be read as regarding the process of labelling as actually causing such phenomena as mental disorder. Moreover, no matter what the original effect of stereotypical attitudes is towards, for example, people with mental disorder, it can be argued that this will be relatively transitory given the occurrence of other more positive actions and images. Furthermore, most people will in any case never enter the secondary stage of labelling (Gove, 1980).

Some, however, have attempted to adjust social reaction theory in order to compensate for its acknowledged weaknesses. Link et al. (1989), for example, have produced what they described as a 'modified labelling theory' for mental disorder in which an attempt is made to avoid the problem of aetiology but still acknowledge the damaging effects of stigma. These authors developed their amended theory through a study of residents ($n = 429$) and psychiatric patients ($n = 164$) in one locality of New York.

What these authors argued was that mentally disordered patients had, on entry to hospital, already been inculcated with negative beliefs about their condition. Thus, the patient colludes with the stigmatized version of mental disorder by performing in ways that confirm the prevailing (negative) imagery. The belief of mentally disordered patients that, when confronted by members of their community, they will be devalued and discriminated against if their disorder is discovered, leads to secretive behaviour and a withdrawal from situations in which they fear they will be rejected. This, suggest Link et al., will lead to further social isolation, unemployment and the loss of self-esteem.

Moral panic

It is widely acknowledged that this is the age of moral panic. Newspaper headlines continually warn of some new danger resulting from moral laxity, and television programmes echo the theme with sensational documentaries. (Thompson, 1998, p1)

For Stanley Cohen (1972), who can be considered as having played the primary role in developing this theory in the UK, the panic is 'moral' because there is a challenge to the ethically acceptable social order. Moreover, those doing the challenging are considered to be morally corrupt to the point of being evil; they are, in his terms, construed as 'folk devils'.

The term 'moral panic' is defined as:

the alleged over-reaction of the mass media, the police and local community leaders to the activities of particular social groups which are in fact *relatively trivial*, both in terms of the nature of the offence and the number of people involved. (Abercrombie et al., 1994, p272–3, original emphasis).

Overstatement and distortion are, therefore, central to the thesis of moral panic. In particular, it is argued, the media engage in what has been described as 'deviancy amplification' (Wilkins, 1964). Once set in motion, a corrupt and stereotypical description of young people, black men, AIDS sufferers, single mothers, Moslem fundamentalists or the mentally disordered results in a helical process of increased embellishment.

Kenneth Thompson (1998) traces the history of moral panic. He describes a century of public alarm over such issues as crime, the leisure habits of young people and the 1960s 'sexual revolution'. For Thompson in later years, however, the nature of moral panic has changed in two ways. First, he argues that moral panics are occurring more frequently and often overlap each other. Second, he suggests that there is now a qualitative difference between earlier panics and present ones:

> Almost anything can spark off a panic, so the initial event can range from something as serious as children killing another child (the murder, in 1993, of James Bulger) to an incident of school bullying; at one time there is a fear about being wiped out by the AIDS epidemic, then there is outrage about the discovery of pornography on the Internet ... Earlier panics tended to be focused on a single group – teenagers who went to coffee bars, drug addicts or young black muggers. Contemporary panics seem to catch more people in their net. For example, panics about child abuse seem to call into question the very institution of the family. (Thompson, 1998, p2)

Thompson identifies the process involved in the development of a moral panic. There is a 'crusade' by, for example, a newspaper editor about a particular social issue. This is then taken up by those who are already alarmed at, and feeling in danger from, what is perceived to be a disintegration of society's moral order. This may be related to a specific and localized threat. For example, inner-city areas with high levels of immigrants and crime may produce anxiety in the 'host' population, which then is given direction and apparent validity when the media reports on street robberies carried out by 'black muggers'. With reference to the mentally disordered, a homicide by a person described in the press as a 'dangerous psychopath' foments and gives focus to an existing concern by people living in urban areas about vagrancy, begging and drunkenness. As a consequence, all members of the targeted group have much more hostility directed towards them than is merited by the crime committed by one person.

Next, the media-initiated campaign is adopted by politicians for a combination of reasons (ranging from unadulterated self-interest to a genuine response to the concerns of their constituents). There are calls for a return to the (probably mythical) morality of a bygone age. Last, there is the realization by those who have conducted the crusade that what they consider to be the key causes of the disordered state of society have not been resolved, and the panic then recedes. Alternatively, some degree of social change ensues. The latter may result in new policies or laws. Alarm over madness and murder has indeed led to changes in both policy and mental health legislation.

However, where policies and laws are introduced, there is, observes Thompson, a lack of clarity concerning what behaviours should or should not be tolerated, or the 'moral' over-reaction is compounded by overzealous policing. In both Britain and the USA, for example, a number of cities have operated a policy of 'zero tolerance' on crime whereby no matter how small the misdemeanour, the full force of the law is applied to the culprit. But in other cities in these countries, the same act will attract no police response whatsoever. Moreover, prostitution and drug addiction are accepted in parts of Britain, and in some senses are 'encouraged' by the supplying of condoms and drugs by some local authorities to prostitutes and addicts. In other regions of Britain, however, these deviant behaviours are vigorously suppressed by the police and local councils.

Stanley Cohen, although epistemologically indebted to labelling theory, opened the way for an account to be made of the structural forces (particularly that of social class) that shape outbursts of panic. It was, however, studies of youth culture and mugging by Stuart Hall and his collaborators (using a Marxist perspective) that was to underscore the role of social structure and culture as an explanation for moral panic (Hall & Jefferson, 1976; Hall et al., 1978). For example, the behaviour, dress and expressed values of working-class youth subcultures in the 1970s were seen to signify the rejection and subversion of the dominant (capitalist) ideology. The media, seen by these authors to share the values of capitalism, then provided sensationalized images of specific sets of activities (for example, fights between different youth groups, and provocative – sexual, blasphemous or racist – dress and adornments), which sparked off a moral panic.

For Thompson (1998), the importance of the contribution made by Hall and his colleagues to the study of moral panic is not their Marxist analysis, which sees the function of the process of scapegoating particular groups as having been (albeit indirectly) orchestrated by, and in the interests of, the dominant class. He suggests that what have been of greater value are their techniques of deciphering the 'narratives' used by the media that nourish public angst. By the time that news items appear in newspapers and on television, they have gone through an elaborate process of editing involving a series of readjustments and many stages of filtration (Howitt, 1998). The media chooses for its audience what it is important to know about, employs stereotypical and inflammatory words and phrases, and renders 'intelligible' the selected incidents. Moreover, there is, from this perspective, an underlying premise that whatever is written (or indeed verbalized) about any event has the characteristics of all ethnographic accounts. That is, there are a number of perceptual and literary reinterpretations of the original material. Paul Atkinson uses the example of Whyte's classic study of the outdoor (deviant) culture in an Italian slum in the USA:

> When we read an ethnographic monograph – say Street Corner Society (Whyte, 1981) – we are implicated in complex processes of reality construction and reconstruction. That book, with all its vivid and realistic descriptive writing, is not a literal representation of the social situation of Italian-American street-corner gang members. Whyte's craft resides not just in the conscientious and careful collection of data, and their arrangement into a factual report. The monograph itself is, in the best sense, an artful product. The narratives and descriptions, the example, the characters and the interpretative commentary are woven together in a highly contrived product. (Atkinson, 1990, p2)

Atkinson also points to further reinterpretations, but this time by the reader of the text. That is, the written word (or visual image) is translated into forms that fit into our own experience-based perceptions and bio-psycho capabilities.

According to Hall and his fellow Marxists, collusion between the ruling class in society and media representations of reality occurs through the delivery of ideologically biased messages from the powerful to newspapers and television. There is, for example, a continuous passage of information from political sources feeding the media. I have to express some surprise at my own discovery, having tapped into the DoH's Internet site, of how newspapers precisely reiterate government press releases. Information about crime, inevitably slanted towards the goals and values of the powerful, is in the main provided by the institutions of the state – the police, judges and the Home Office.

The concept of 'hegemony', introduced into Marxist thought by Antonio Gramsci, is utilized by Hall et al. (1978). Gramsci (1891–1937), an Italian communist militant imprisoned for 10 years by Mussolini, was one of the most influential Marxist thinkers of the twentieth century. Hegemony, for Gramsci (1971), is the way in which the dominant class suffuses the values of the individual (who may belong to another social class and thereby have competing beliefs) with its own ideological predispositions. Through a myriad of indoctrinating processes, we come to accept as 'common sense' the ideas of right and wrong that work to support the interests of this dominant group.

The implication here is that the moral panic in Britain in the 1970s about 'black muggers' was an example of the ruling class 'using' Afro-Caribbean men in its ideological campaign to readjust social values away from the extravagancies of the 1960s and towards law and order. Moral panic, therefore, becomes an ideological conduit, giving notice of what behaviours will and will not be tolerated.

Thompson (1998) suggests that the political establishment and media have a vested interest in the manufacture of moral panics that is not merely ideological, but also pragmatic. Put simply, the media need audiences, and experience has shown editors of newspapers, and television and radio producers, that sensationalizing a story and demonizing certain players in that story increases the size of the audience. Politicians can also concentrate on moral issues rather than provide answers to intractable social problems such as unemployment, poverty and crime. A moral panic with a target group whose vote is insubstantial will, of course, be particularly convenient.

This view of self-interest by the media and politicians in relation to moral panics is endorsed by Angela McRobbie and Sarah Thornton in their influential article 'Rethinking "moral panic" for multimediated social worlds' (1995). McRobbie & Thornton suggest that creating alarm in the public domain through the media is directly linked to commerce. Terrorizing readers and viewers not only sells newspapers, and provides high ratings for television and radio programmes, but also 'advertises' certain products. These authors cite the example of how record companies promoted a brand of music called 'acid house' in the 1980s. The record companies claimed that the music was controversial in that it was associated with the promotion of drug use. The media duly decried it as 'outrageous'. Marketed as such, young people were fairly certain to take an interest.

There is, however, disagreement over the claim by moral panic theorists that the response by the media is disproportionate to the threat (Thompson, 1998). The question here is, 'Can the reaction of journalists and the community to, for example, certain types of crime ever be regarded as warranted?' In Stuart Hall and his colleagues' work (Hall et al., 1978) on mugging, it is avowed that an irrational and exaggerated response by the media and the public to 'black muggers' was generated (or at least not suppressed) by the ruling class. This was done, argue Hall et al., to prevent attention being attracted to the economic and cultural difficulties that the capitalist system was at that point undergoing. This thesis has, however, been criticized for not acknowledging the actual increase in urban crime happening at the time (Waddington, 1986). That is, Waddington argues that Hall et al. misrepresented the real level of crime and the understandable effect on, and reaction by, the white working class in inner-city areas. It is also somewhat ironic – and contradictory – that Marxists at root accept the positivistic notion of there being an objective reality (a reality that will be 'revealed' following the unveiling of the 'mystifying' ideology of capitalism), but Hall et al. adopt constructionist thought in their critique of the media. Constructionism is antagonistic to beliefs in objective reality.

A revision of moral panic theory has been presented by McRobbie & Thornton (1995). These authors highlight the fact that it has been decades since deviancy theory spawned the moral panic approach, and important changes have been occurring in media technology and in the way in which advocates for vulnerable groups operate. McRobbie & Thornton argue that the media has become more influential and diverse in the industrialized world, and that there has been vigorous campaigning by lobbyists. This, they argue, has resulted in a watering-down of folk-devil imagery. Campaign experts are now recruited by interest groups to perpetuate the views of these groups and to respond immediately to any adverse publicity in the media. In an ideological war of manoeuvre, these experts embark on a counterattack if under fire from journalists and politicians.

Rapid-response advocacy certainly exists in the mental health industry. Survey work by MIND, the British mental health charity, has provided evidence of continued discrimination towards the mentally disordered in many areas of civil life (Reed & Baker, 1996; Repper et al., 1997). This ranges from difficulties in gaining insurance policies to a persistent and pervasive occurrence of 'nimbyism' ('not in my backyard') by local communities when faced with the prospect of mentally disturbed neighbours. The following quotation, from the general manager of a local user organization, refers to the backlash from the community when it was discovered that a group home was being established:

> It was last summer, a short time before users were due to go in. The van outside was plastered with slogans like 'schizophrenics go home', the fence and the house was daubed with paint and abuse. (Repper et al., 1997, p3)

Within its wider 'Respect' campaign, aimed at countering prejudicial perceptions and structural inequality, MIND is (quite understandably) blatantly in favour of media spin-doctoring. For example, in an information leaflet from the campaign, it declares an intention to:

> have created [by 1999] a measurable shift in media coverage, with less 'mad axeman' and stereotpyed coverage, and more examples which illuminate the different realities of people's lives. (Sayce, 1997, p3)

The strategies that MIND promotes to ensure that these 'different realities' hold sway involve: developing methods of working with schools to educate the young about mental health issues and prejudice; informing employers of their obligations under the Disability Discrimination Act 1995, and assisting them to make adjustments in their working environment so that the high unemployment levels amongst the long-term mentally disordered can be reduced; and providing guidance to health services about how to deal with apprehensive local communities.

More specifically with regard to the role of the media, there seems to be a tacit acceptance by MIND of postmodernist notions of 'hyperreality'. That is, as Jean Baudrillard (1981, 1983, 1988) has argued, that the media does not simply relay reality – or even representations of reality – to its audience, but is engaged in projecting a simulated world. For Baudrillard, therefore, social events have become 'objects for manipulation'. Certainly, MIND's tactics appear to include the 'reorganization' of conventional imagery. For example, MIND states a commitment to:

> work with other mental health organisations to influence commissioning editors, as well as inspiring positive programmes and articles on mental health issues; support and train users in making decisions about whether to go public to the media about their experiences; and collaborate with well-known people who may want to 'come out' as users ... Work with the local media to promote positive examples of users' lives. (Sayce, 1997, p4)

McRobbie & Thornton comment that lobbyism has coincided with the state's measures to ensure control becoming less resolute. The suggestion is that the state now operates an incohesive and faltering system of social control, and cannot therefore be sure of successfully and consistently using the scapegoating of particular groups as a method of maintaining the *status quo*. However, McRobbie & Thornton's recognition of the commercial imperative behind some forms of moral panic also implies that the state, although undoubtedly mutating in response to the cultural, political and economic vagaries of late-modernity, maintains its inherent capitalist ideological orientation. Moreover, this must be as a consequence of techniques of social control remaining effective and profound. Hegemony is never complete (Hazelton, 1995), but the dominance of the ruling class remains both secure and persistent.

McRobbie & Thornton point out that the media often contain contradictory and hypocritical stances. For example, a newspaper or television station may be indignant about a social or health problem, but accommodate explicit or surreptitious 'advertisements' for commodities associated with generating that problem. This has happened consistently with regard to smoking, drug abuse and environmental pollution. There is nothing unusual in finding that a television production about the effects of cancer or liver transplants, or

the toxic effects on children of high lead levels in the air, is followed
by commercials for alcohol and cars, or a soap opera in which large
amounts of alcohol and tobacco are consumed. Furthermore, whilst
emphatically taking a high moral position on an issue, the media
may be actively and knowingly titillating its readership. McRobbie &
Thornton use the example of the British tabloid newspaper the *Sun*,
which is seen to be impassioned in its moralizing:

> With a topless sixteen year old on page 3 and a hedonistic pro-sex editorial
> line ... that doesn't stop them from being the most preachy and prescriptive
> of Britain's daily papers, with page after page of the '*Sun* says...' However,
> the *Sun*'s favourite moral panics are of the 'sex, drugs and rock'n'roll' variety
> – stories about other people having far *too much* fun ... Moreover, these kinds
> of story have the advantage of allowing their readers to have their cake and
> eat it too; they can vicariously enjoy and/or secretly admire the transgres-
> sion one moment, then be shocked and offended the next. (McRobbie &
> Thornton, 1995, p569, original emphasis)

Moreover, the effect of moral panics may be more convoluted
than simply causing misery to those people who have been singled
out for blame. For example, overstating the threat to society of
particular groups or events can be counterproductive. Propelling
'glue sniffing', 'under-age sex' or 'football hooliganism' onto the
front pages of newspapers and into the lead items of news broadcasts
may encourage more people to be attracted to these activities, especially where detailed accounts are provided. Furthermore, where
deviancy is the consequence of marginalization, punitive laws
designed to castigate severely those who have caused such outrage
may force the culprits to become more isolated and therefore much
less likely to be rehabilitated.

McRobbie & Thornton record another paradox regarding
media accounts of 'the facts'. This time it is within moral panic
theory itself. The critical stance taken by social scientists who use
moral panic theory to accuse the media of exaggeration are intu-
itively accepting that truth can be found.

Postmodern impostures

In the postmodern rendition of constructionism, however, truth has
been utterly abandoned. Postmodern thinkers have pronounced that

the late twentieth century produced a pattern of pluralistic and frag-
mented lifestyles, whereby there is now no longer any overarching
political, legal, moral or epistemological authority to be found in
society (Lyotard, 1984). The 'grand narratives' of, for example,
nationhood, Christianity, socialism, the free market, science and the
law have disappeared, or are acclaimed by only a minority of the
population. There is, therefore, no one way of comprehending either
the social or the physical world. Moreover, there has been a demise
in the degree of deference formerly shown to leaders, experts, teachers, the police and the judiciary.

But at the same there is frenzied consumerism, which causes all
aspects of life (from food to sexuality) to be reconstrued as commodities, and a polarization of people into two social arenas – 'the
wealthy employed' and the impoverished 'underclass'. These trends,
when combined with the loss of unifying authoritative control, have
the effect of further alienating the dispossessed and of fomenting
disorder (Reiner, 1997).

Therefore, the 'problem' of crime is not a problem as such but a
manifestation of the 'postmodern condition', the consequence of
what Zygmunt Bauman (1997) views as the inescapable messiness of
the human predicament. There are, however, no logical recipes or
rational solutions to be found to this messiness. There may be
temporary answers to specific issues, but a permanent resolution of
all or any of the anxieties and uncertainties that occur for individuals
or society is not possible. We have to live with ambiguity, social
discordance and our discontents.

Furthermore, the postmodern 'deconstruction' of all cultural
phenomena as merely the outcome of various discursive practices,
and the view that social and physical life is 'constructed' in every
respect, leaves crime without any validity as a 'social fact'. In this
sense, postmodernist thinking is commensurate with the social reaction and moral panic theorists' standpoint that deviancy is nothing
more than behaviour that has come to be labelled as unacceptable
by those groups in society with the power so to do (Lea, 1998).

Although by no means a postmodernist, Thomas Szasz's proposition that madness is an invention, based on the literal and inappropriate use of 'illness' as a metaphor for everyday problems,
exemplifies the postmodern position on this form of deviancy. More-

over, in his examination of court processes, Szasz deconstructs the category of homicidal insanity, claiming that it is purely a tag of convenience. Homicidal insanity, comments Szasz, is a label that is purposefully adopted by the killer's defence lawyer, with the aid of psychiatric opinion:

> (so-called) psychotics assert that they hear voices that command them to kill their wives or children; psychiatrists assert that such persons suffer from a brain disease called 'schizophrenia', which can be effectively treated with certain chemicals; and I claim that the assertions of psychotics and psychiatrists alike are claims unsubstantiated by evidence ... after shooting his wife, the killer's court appointed lawyer, desperate to 'defend' him (perhaps against his nominal client's wishes), claims that the illegal act was caused by schizophrenia and that the killer should therefore be 'acquitted' and treated in a mental hospital, rather than punished by imprisonment. (Szasz, 1994, pp37–8)

Postmodern accounts of criminology can be seen as so fatalistic that it may seem to justify the non-criminal population having to just accept a rising crime rate. On the other hand, the absence of any sustainable moral code can presumably offer emancipation for victims as well as offenders, thereby allowing those belonging to the 'polarized rich' to protect themselves, their homes and their work environments:

> For those in society who can afford it, provision of security will be increasingly privatized, either in residential areas or the 'mass private property' where more and more middle-class leisure and work takes place. (Reiner, 1997, p1039)

Moreover, new technologies for monitoring public spaces (for example, closed-circuit television) are being used extensively to safeguard property and consumers. Added to this is the employment of sophisticated surveillance and control techniques aimed at the underclass and deviants. Health visitors monitor the behaviour of single mothers, and the psychopath who is considered to be 'potentially' dangerous (and who invariably belongs to the lowest part of the social hierarchy) is incarcerated in a secure unit. These measures will allow the interests of the middle-class citizen, powerful professional groups and the state to endure even in the chaos of postmodern life.

But to argue that crime is a dependent variable of social control policies, cultural variations, labelling or media attention underplays (or even discounts altogether) the effect of crime on those victims who cannot protect themselves. Declaring that causes of crime are the result of certain sections of the population being scapegoated by, for example, the police and the courts is of little compensation when we are robbed in the street, our houses are burgled or our cars are stolen. The victims of these particular crimes can of course be gratified that a low prosecution rate avoids the stigmatization of offenders.

Alan Sokal (Professor of physics at New York University) and Jean Bricmont (Professor of theoretical physics at the University of Louvain in Belgium) have taken it upon themselves to 'deconstruct' a number of the central tenets of postmodernist thought. Their project has been to attack what they see as a misreading and mistreatment of scientific propositions, and the intellectual posturing and blatant dishonesty of prominent postmodernists. Specifically, Sokal & Bricmont assail the foundation of postmodernist thinking – epistemological relativism – which regards science as a social construction and therefore merely one 'truth' amongst many other possible truths.

Their quest follows the famous spoof conducted by Sokal whereby he sent a largely nonsensical 'postmodernist' article to a leading American cultural-studies journal (*Social Text*) and had it published. In a convincing and devastating critique of works by Jacques Lacan, Luce Irigaray, Bruno Latour, Gilles Deleuze and Jean Baudrillard, Sokal & Bricmont conclude that social scientists should not study what they do not understand (that is, science).

With reference to criminology, these authors provide an example of the absurd position in which those with postmodernist tendencies can place themselves with respect to the 'truth'. They record the case in Belgium of the murder of children in 1996 and the perceived ineptitude of the police investigation. During a televised session conducted by a parliamentary commission, two witnesses (one a police officer and the other a judge) contested each other's versions of what had happened to an important file. The policeman's story was that he had sent the file to the judge, but the latter claimed not to have received it. On the following day, a senior academic in the field of 'communication' was interviewed for a leading Belgium newspaper. The journalist conducting the interview, referring to the discrepancy between what the two witnesses had said about the file, asked whether or not the academic believed in 'truth'. The academic responded that there are only 'partial truths' that are shared by groups of people, and that both of the witnesses were 'telling the truth'. Sokal & Bricmont observe:

> The dispute between the policeman and the judge concerns after all, material fact: the transmission of a file. (It is of course possible that the file was sent but lost on the way; but this remains a well-defined factual question.) Without a doubt, the epistemological problem is complicated: how is the commission to find out what really happened? Nevertheless, there *is* a truth of the matter: either the file was sent or it wasn't. (Sokal & Bricmont, 1998, p92, original emphasis).

One is left to wonder whether or not the same relativist submission could have been applied to the murder of the children. Perhaps no-one was really 'guilty' of the crime, and maybe the children were not really dead as 'living' is a 'truth' that is as open to interpretation as whether or not a file was sent from one person to another.

John Lea (1998) argues that the most obvious defect in the post-modernist's desire to 'deconstruct' everything is that of 'infinite regress'. If social and physical phenomena are shown to not be what they seem, what they become (after having been deconstructed) can also be decomposed *ad infinitum*:

> The fact that we never arrive – and from a postmodern standpoint must not arrive – at any sort of rock bottom concepts that we can say 'really' describe an external reality means that methods such as deconstruction lead to infinite regress. Deconstruction is like spending time with a dictionary looking up words that are defined in terms of other words, which can in turn be looked up and so on. (Lea, 1998, pp169–70)

For example, the deconstruction of 'madness' may produce a novel comprehension of psychotic behaviour as an 'existential', 'phenomenological' or 'spiritual' state of being. However, these reconstituted understandings will also be susceptible to the same process of degeneration of given meanings that destroyed the original interpretation. How then can the suffering of the mad be addressed or even recognized as being legitimate and in need of succour? Presumably, both the idea of suffering and the concept of legitimacy are liable to deconstruction.

Summary

The contribution of the constructionist theorists to the study of criminality and madness has been to establish the relativity of behaviour (that is, the meaning given to an action is dependent upon alterable perceptions), to place centre stage the concept of 'social control' in the organization of deviant classifications, and to highlight how the reaction of powerful groups in society affects the process of labelling and stigmatization. However, neither labelling theory nor the perspective of moral panic can explain the original cause of criminality or mental disorder. Both can be accused of offering sustenance to the offender and deviant whilst ignoring the distress of others as a result of their actions. The social actor within these approaches is portrayed as reacting mechanically to such external influences as the media, unable to resist the implanting of an identity foreign to his or her present self-image.

Moreover, the attachment of 'stigma' could be regarded as a necessary stabilizing measure that controls those behaviours which would otherwise damage the individual and the community. The stigma of mental disorder may well be less severe in its consequences for the individual than, for example, imprisonment or ignoring his or her psychological torment.

The contribution of postmodern deliberations is, however, much less equivocal. Postmodernists are intellectual 'impostures'. Their depositions are fallacious and impenetrable, the conceptualization of the human condition and the physical environment an ingenuous contrivance, their campaign to 'deconstruct everything' an example of naive nihilism. Few, if any, profitable insights into madness and murder can be gained from such cerebral masturbation.

Chapter 7
Get real

The critical analysis of the three 'fault-driven' criminological taxonomies offered in Chapters 4, 5 and 6 has pointed to a conglomeration of factors that need to be introduced into the debate about what causes crime and deviancy, and what can be done about the problem of antisocial behaviour. This analysis has, however, also demonstrated that each explanatory framework on its own has irredeemable shortcomings.

The resolution, I suggest, is to be found within the speculations of 'realist theory'. Realist theory provides a synthesis of the positivist-constructionist 'knowledge' dichotomy found in the preceding genres. In doing so, it rehabilitates human verve regarding the 'problem of crime' and grants the actuality of madness and murder.

Reflexive reality

The positions taken by the protagonists of rationalist social contract theory and scientific positivism, social positivism and constructionism, are inadequate. To lay blame for legal and social transgressions on the innate irresponsibility or pathology of the individual, the structural dimensions of the capitalist mode of production and patriarchy, or labelling processes and the media, reduces humans to prostrate objects. Within these accounts, the behaviour of the human actor is determined by his or her psycho-biological constitution, evolution, the social environment or the 'constructs' of the powerful.

Moreover, the 'problem of crime' then becomes prone to the theoretical vagaries derived from natural science, social science and politics. The way in which crime is conceptualized and how it is tackled sways, depending on, for example, the discovery of new 'criminal' genes or the unravelling of Darwinian-based traits, the further deconstruction of 'false' labels or which governmental doctrine happens to be in vogue.

The implication of realism, however, is that the human actor is both shaped by and helps to shape his or her social world. That is, humans have a reflexive relationship not just with each other, but also with society. What an individual does and thinks affects the content and form of social processes and the way in which society is structured. Equally, social processes and structures configure the circumstances in which human actions and cognition can operate. However, neither the 'human condition' nor the social system remains static. Both change in ways that make their effect on each other difficult to predict.

Reflexivity does not mean that there are no facts, or that those facts which are heavily laden with social meaning do not have actual and legitimate significance for those involved, but it is accepted by realists that a knowledge of what is a 'fact' can only be approximated. Madness and murder are examples of social phenomena that retain ambiguity as categories, are generously impregnated with cultural meaning and are difficult to define, but are not *ipso facto* mere abstractions or metaphors. Moreover, realist theorists observe that crime is a reality that affects the vulnerable (for example, the working class, women, children and ethnic minorities). Therefore, for realists, crime needs to be confronted and contained (Young, 1986). Furthermore, realism argues that those who suffer from the acts of criminals should not simply accept their 'victim' role. That is, potential and actual victims of crime are not impotent recipients of bio-psycho and social forces, on whom harm is done but from whom nothing can be expected in terms of altering the world in which they exist. Individuals, collectivities (such as neighbours on a housing estate) and the community as a whole can fight back against the impositions of criminality on the quality of life.

The perspective of 'realism' can be read as not only vituperative of positivistic approaches and social reaction/moral panic theorists, but also most specifically an attack on the extreme relativism of postmodernist accounts of the social and physical world (Clarke & Layder, 1994). The profound scepticism of the postmodernist critique leads to a destruction of faith in objective reality and a mistrust of established knowledge. Universal values - be they religious, political or economic – are no longer perceived to be tenable or credible except in the sense that 'anything goes' (including previous 'truths') as far as styles of living are concerned. What we take as 'normal' and 'moral' is only meaningful and 'right' within the historical and cultural context in which it occurs. For the postmodernist, therefore, there are no licit assurances about how to behave in any aspect of our social and personal lives. Facts and certainties are unobtainable (Lawson & Appignananesi, 1989).

However, the realist position on knowledge, as on human action, is reflexive in substance. Whilst attacking as credulous both the objectivism of natural science and the subjectivism of constructionism and postmodernism, its proponents see a mutuality between empirical facts and how humans interpret their world:

> Realists suggest that social analysis should include both underlying (and to some extent unobservable) social phenomena, without rejecting the importance of subjective experience. (Layder, 1994, p45)

By rejecting the standard antithetical positions of positivism (searching for an objective reality) and constructionism (reality is the result of subjective interpretation), realism in a sense offers a 'third way' in epistemology. However, rather than going down the postmodernist path of epistemological self-destruction, whereby all knowledge is susceptible to deconstruction and all human action is (relatively) meaningful to individuals, groups and cultures but has also no 'essential' meaning, realism reinterprets human understanding of the material and social world. That is, the relationship between epistemology (how we know what we know) and ontology (what we consider we are as humans) is redefined as having both objective and subjective qualities (Morrow, 1994). Scientific methods can offer (some) insights into what we understand our existence to be, but human intuition, introspection and experience also contribute to 'knowledge'.

Critical realism

It is the 'critical' realism of Roy Bhaskar (1986, 1989, 1997, 1998) that has produced a coming together of 'factual' and 'constructed' knowledge:

men in their social activity produce knowledge which is a social product
much like any other, which is no more independent of its production and the
men who produce it than motor cars, armchairs or books, which has its own
craftsmen, technicians, publicists, standards and skills, and which is not less
subject to change than any other commodity. This is one side of 'knowledge'. The other is that knowledge is '*of*' things which are not produced by
men at all: the specific gravity of mercury, the process of electrolysis, the
mechanism of light propagation. None of these 'objects of knowledge'
depend upon human activity. If men ceased to exist sound would continue
to travel and heavy bodies to fall to the earth in exactly the same way.
(Bhaskar, 1998, p16, original emphasis)

For Bhaskar, what we experience as objective reality can be
viewed as contingent upon the relative values of our cultural and
temporal existence, but this does mean that knowable and concrete
realities cannot be found. We are, however, according to Bhaskar,
restricted in our ability to know these realities because of the
inevitable limitations imposed on us by the culture to which we
belong and the contaminated and inept methods used by science to
detect objective realities. Put simply, there are concrete objects and
universal laws, but humans can only experience these subjectively
and can, therefore, never 'know', in the purest sense, anything.
Science offers us a 'best guess' of what these objects are and how the
world operates.

The continuous rearranging and updating of scientific knowledge (and at times complete paradigm shifts), as well as the frequent
publishing of contrary research findings, can be seen to be a consequence of the trouble that humans have identifying inaccurately the
causes of physical and social phenomena. Cognitive mechanisms
and intracultural norms 'mystify' reality – but, for Bhaskar, there is
actually a reality to be mystified!

For Bhaskar, 'intransitive knowledge' (the invariable 'facts' that
exist with or without our knowledge of them) can only be mediated
through 'transitive knowledge' (the vocabulary, concepts and technologies of the 'science' of the day). That is, scientific endeavour is
about investigating and attempting to disclose the real structures,
processes, mechanisms and events of the world through the use of
preceding understandings and predictions. For example, the discovery of how blood circulates in the human body by the English physician William Harvey (1578–1657) required a model of hydraulics
that had been handed down from ancient times and modified

throughout the intervening period. Contemporary notions of, and treatment for, madness are the result of a process of medicalization stemming from the successful take-over of the asylums by practitioners of physical medicine in the eighteenth and nineteenth centuries. Present-day legal and moral adjudication on killing has a Judaeo-Christian heritage founded over the previous two millennia.

Furthermore, society functions relatively well in the province of this approximated reality. Most of us live perfectly purposefully in this part-virtual world, unaware that what we embrace as substance is somewhat flaky. It would seem that we have an indelible and unconscious appetite to conjure up a solid world of matter, to 'make sense' of what we see around us despite frequent contradictions and paradoxical data. We are, in the main, instinctive pragmatists, with only the mad (and postmodernists) experiencing the high level of ontological insecurity that accompanies insight into the indeterminancy of the external world.

Gerald Delanty (1997), however, points out that there has been a misreading of the constructionist project. He attempts to reconcile constructionism with realism. In order to produce a theoretical tract 'beyond' that of either constructionist or realist approaches, Delanty argues that both in essence (apart from the extravagant claims of those who believe that there has been a complete dissolution of 'truth') accept reality. However, they differ in how much stress should be placed on reality in shaping knowledge, social events and relationships:

> Except for extreme constructivism [i.e. postmodernism], constructivists do not deny the existence of social reality as an objective entity. The stress, in general, is on how social actors construct their reality ... Realists, unlike constructivists, *emphasize* that realities underlying knowledge do exist. (Delanty, 1997, p129, emphasis added)

There is, therefore, for Delanty, a 'false dichotomy' between constructionism and realism, but it is the very nature of the constructionist underplay of reality that makes the difference significant. That is, the contribution of realism to the critique of both positivism and constructionism is to recognize the collusion between 'facts' and social processes. It is this intermingling of the actual and the social that gives realism its dynamism and makes it distinct from positivism and constructionism.

'New left' realism

This understanding of the reflexive relationship between individuals and society, and the collusion between facts and social processes, has been applied to criminology by the 'new left realism' (NLR) of Jock Young, Roger Mathews and John Lea. These authors, with their proclaimed mandate of 'taking crime seriously' and of having criminology theory 'policy-relevant', have introduced a number of innovations to the analysis of crime (Lea & Young, 1984; Mathews & Young, 1986; Young & Mathews, 1992).

For example, NLR posits (against positivism) that it is impossible to make 'factual' generalizations about the aetiology of crime. To suggest that individual pathology or unemployment leads to crime ignores the huge variation in types of crime. That is, one single factor cannot be seen to cause rape, tax fraud, violence against the person and traffic offences. For the theorists of NLR, however, complaints by women that they feel intimidated at night in the inner-city areas, the fears of the elderly about burglary, the existence of domestic violence and racist assaults must be accepted as the legitimate concerns of individuals and communities (Young, 1986). Although accepting that there is always a danger that certain collections of people may be scapegoated and declared 'folk devils', Young (1986) argues that much of what is expressed by vulnerable sections of the population is credible. Young acknowledges that 'fear displacement' and 'tunnel vision' affect perceptions of crime, but he cites the example of the under-reporting of sexual attacks to suggest not only that public fears have a basis in reality, but also that even more of an outcry than has already occurred may be warranted.

The supporters of an extreme version of 'moral panic' theory, which views the 'problem of crime' purely as the result of media attention (for example, Chambliss, 1994; Platt, 1996), are attacked by Young. Reflecting upon the origins of moral panic theory (in which Young had an involvement during its development), he refers to the levels of violence within the black community and homicide overall in the USA to illustrate the absurdity of the way in which the theory has been applied by these authors:

> To talk of moral panic about crime in the United States beggars the imagi-
> nation and trivializes a concept which was introduced to contrast the panic

about minor offences (e.g. cannabis or mods fighting on Brighton beaches)
with real problems of crime ... I have already documented the appalling
figures within the African-American community, so high that a recent radical researcher writes that it is 'a form of black genocide, since the victim of
homicide is most often another black person and the incidence of this crime
is so pervasive' (Mann, 1993, p.46). Are these writers really suggesting that
there is a moral panic about black crime. And even the general rate is stag-
geringly high: the number of homicides, for example, in Los Angeles with a
population of 3.5 million, is greater than that of England and Wales with
over fifty million inhabitants. (Young, 1997, p478)

Young makes the point that, with this background of violence
and murder, it would be astonishing if the public were not somewhat
agitated and were unconcerned about the morality of the criminal
activity that they experience at first hand. Central to the realist position is an acknowledgement of the fear of crime as having a rational
basis. People get scared because there is something to be scared
about. That is, there is an understandable and rational core of fear.
Crime exists and hurts people and communities.

Jock Young and his realist collaborators' position on the relationship between the social order and crime could be condemned as
reactionary in the sense that the issue of crime is being addressed
pragmatically. Young, however, places NLR firmly in the radical
dimension of criminology. That is, although 'realistic' about crime,
he accepts that the effect of inequalities in capitalist society (particularly those produced by poverty and patriarchy) cannot be ignored.
Therefore, for Young (1997), NLR is not an 'establishment' criminology. Crime is not a social 'blemish' that can be eviscerated, leav-
ing an otherwise healthy society. Capitalist society is, for Young, with
its investment in individual competitiveness and male dominance
and aggression, in need of reconstruction:

> The solution is to be found not in the resurrection of past stabilities, based on
> nostalgia and a world that will never return, but on a new citizenship, a
> reflexive modernity which will tackle the problems of justice and commu-
> nity, of reward and individualism, which dwell at the heart of liberal democ-
> racy. (Young, 1999, p199)

Young (1997) traces the political context of the origins of NLR.
It was developed in response to the rise of 'punishment-orientated'
policies towards crime put in place in the 1980s by right-wing

governments such as that of Margaret Thatcher in Britain. Deterrent strategies in the criminal justice system were the other side of the raging individualism created by the market-driven political and economic strategies of the right. Although not admitting a causal relationship, a reduction in commitment from the governments of the right to the welfare state, and worker participation in the organization of industry, alongside a deliberate policy of massively increasing unemployment (in order to raise competitiveness by reducing wages), coincided with a huge upsurge in the crime rate. The right's answer was to declare its allegiance to the law-abiding majority and to build more prisons.

At the time, according to Young, the response of left-wing and liberal theorists and politicians was a mirror image of the right-wing approach. That is, the left seemed hell-bent on denying that there was a problem of crime and on portraying the offender in the role of victim. The left was accused, in promoting (or waiting for) extensive social change, of being idealistic and Utopian, and of being irresponsible for not tackling crime and the effects of crime, much of which was detrimental to the quality of lives of those whom the left purported to represent – the working class.

Hence, the criminal justice system, far from performing only in the interests of the élite classes (and, therefore, from the perspective of the left beyond redemption), could and should be mandated to protect the working class.

For Young, there needed to be a pathway found between these two antagonistic political routes. The maxim for this middle course became 'take crime seriously':

> The springboard for the emergence of realist criminology was the injunction to 'take crime seriously', an urgent recognition that crime was a real problem for a large section of the population, particularly women, the most vulnerable sections of the working class, and the ethnic minorities. It emerged as a critique of a predominant tendency in left wing and liberal commentaries which downplayed the problem of crime, *talking about media instigated moral panics and irrational fears of crime*. (Young, 1997, p474, emphasis added)

Realists point to the primacy of deprivation and its consequences (that is, discontent) in the cause of crime (Young, 1998, 1999). Young, in an attempt to avoid going towards absolutist versions of social determinism, argues that there is no evidence (using such measures as unemployment, overcrowding and poor educational opportunities) that deprivation causes crime in any linear way. That is, crime can occur in any part of society and at any time. The absence of wealth and/or low social position as such is not a major cause of crime. Most poor people do not, and many wealthy people do, commit crimes. On the other hand, crime and deviancy are 'everywhere'; but it is posited by the realists that 'relative' deprivation is the key to understanding the aetiology of crime.

However, although relative deprivation breeds dissatisfaction, crime is most likely to be the outcome if a lack of resources is combined with the politics of individualism and gross marginalization. The adverse consequences of individualistic self-expression and self-interest demanded by a market-led economy are, for Young (1998), crime and villainy. But the individual is not simply driven to crime by these factors: he or she still makes a conscious choice over whether or not to indulge in criminal activity:

> Human discontent is experience, by evaluation, by judgement of fairness and just allocation. It is not about simple economic deficit ... Thus the path from social injustice to crime is mediated by human evaluation and the specific possibilities which confront the citizens of a particular society. It is not automatic. (Young, 1999, p159)

Here the realists are indebted to Robert Merton's (1938) concept of 'innovative criminality', discussed in Chapter 5. They argue that where people perceive that they are living in an unjust social system, whereby access to resources and status is unfairly distributed, they will make individual decisions (in a society that discourages communal activity and responsibility) to acquire these valued possessions by other (illegitimate) means. Crime, therefore, occurs more frequently amongst certain sections of society when special conditions come into play – those which are the consequence of an unmeritocratic and 'exclusive society' (Young, 1999).

Young (1997) provides the example of unemployment. He reasons that being unemployed does not mean that an individual will turn to crime. He or she is more prone to be discontented, however, if being unemployed is seen to have arisen from an injustice. This may, for example, have been as a result of, in that person's view, an unfair dismissal, or it could have been prevented by government intervention. The social exclusion and impoverishment that may follow his or her unemployment (particularly if it is long term) will exacerbate the resentment. These factors can, suggest the realists, explain why crime becomes a choice in a situation where other choices are limited. Crime-ridden areas of South Africa may, suggests Young (1998), get even worse if the black population does not receive more tangible outcomes for its aspirations following the destruction of apartheid. Discontent within the major cities in particular will increase the longer it takes for blacks to reach the level of white material accumulation as the discrepancies between both communities remain all too apparent. High rates of homicide in these cities are an indication of the envy and anger that has already marked post-apartheid South Africa.

But crime may occur amongst any social group, in any country and at any time where there is a sense of unjust reward for commensurate effort (Young, 1998, 1999). Crime is more prevalent amongst those at the bottom of the social hierarchy because they are more aggrieved than the middle-classes and the powerful. However, the proliferation of 'white-collar' crime in capitalist society can be viewed as the product of the same factors that contribute to crime of the working class and underclass. That is, the individualism that drives a business executive to extort personal rewards (in the form of money or social advantage) from a commercial deal is likely to be aimed at ensuring his or her acceptance within the higher echelons of the social hierarchy.

In rejecting biological causative factors altogether, Young observes that both the social determinists and the constructionists have thrown the baby out with the bath water. That is, whilst rejecting biological reductionism in the causation of crime, he argues that certain biological elements in the make-up of criminals have to be embraced. Specifically, the realization that there is a correlation between male hormones and violence, and that physically powerful men are far more of a threat than most women, cannot be sidestepped. However, the realist argument is that these biological factors are mediated through social processes. Male violence towards women, and the machismo of working class male youths, is a combination of first, a society based on patriarchy and gender stereotyping, and second, the corporeal disposition of men and women.

For the realist, 'objective facts' (such as evidence of male aggression being affected by biochemicals) must be placed within the relevant cultural or subcultural context. It is the 'lived' reality of the criminal and those touched by crime (especially the victims) that needs to be understood.

Realistic policies

The realist proposition is, however, one of affirming the criminal justice system and the police rather than, as with traditional left-wing approaches, arguing that these operate only as a repressive state apparatus and therefore should not be condoned or should even be abolished. The intention of the realist campaign is to gain greater accountability from the police and to redirect the efforts of the criminal justice system towards offences that hit the working class and underclass, and other vulnerable groups (for example, street crime, male violence towards women and racial harassment). For the realists, there is also a need for 'crimes of the powerful' (for example, political 'sleaze', illegal financial trading by business corporations, and industrial pollution of the environment) to be dealt with effectively by the criminal justice system.

In Young's (1986) terms, 'impossibilism' must be combated. That is, the rising crime rate and high level of recidivism should not lead to a conclusion that 'nothing can be done'. Indeed, this objection to defeatism seems to have had an effect on policy. In the 1990s in Britain, both Conservative and Labour governments announced a crack-down on crime. For example, prime minister Tony Blair, in 1998, pledged an offensive on the activities of criminals. Under the banner of 'order maintenance', structural problems and crime focal points are converged on, and the victims are brought into the picture:

> the Prime Minister today put his personal weight behind the 'zero tolerance' scheme to target 25 towns and cities as crime 'hotspots' ... [The] police are to be asked to adopt a twin track policy of 'order maintenance' – also known as zero tolerance – in crime hotspots ... concentrating police effort on a small area with particular crime problems, and policing it very strictly ... means that thieves, burglars, vandals, and drug-takers are all charged and taken to court when they are arrested, and not just cautioned ... The second tech-

nique to be highlighted by Tony Blair today is based on a very simple idea: that policing should be about solving underlying problems in the community – and not just simply responding to emergency calls. (Hetherington, 1998)

Zero tolerance (or 'order maintenance') is, however, a contentious policy. It was introduced into such cities as New York in the summer of 1994. New York Mayor Rudi Giuliani set out to tackle the immense and historical crime problem by arresting those found indulging in 'low-level' criminal activity. Arresting those committing minor offences involving, for example, prostitution, begging, drugs, driving or vandalism was aimed at preventing further more serious crimes taking place, and thereby allowing the public to enjoy the city's parks and streets without the fear of becoming victims of theft, rape or murder.

Two years after the introduction of zero tolerance into New York, the number of homicides had halved and that of robberies dropped by a third (Chaudhary & Walker, 1996). However, there will have to be a long-term assessment of zero tolerance as a crime policy before a judgement can be made on its efficacy. It may be, for example, inappropriate to export this approach to other countries where esoteric cultural and structural factors could make it inoperable.

Moreover, there is an inevitable down-side to the intense policing of one geographical area (albeit the size of New York city), and that is the stopping, questioning and possibly arresting of a large number of innocent citizens. The law-abiding public may become hostile to the police because of continually coming under suspicion of having committed a misdemeanour, and may refuse to cooperate with the policy. The policy may even be scuppered if those who have been harassed or 'wrongfully arrested' claim damages from the police. Furthermore, Young (1997, 1998, 1999) argues that there cannot be just one strategy for tackling all forms of crime. For Young, not only does there have to be a range of crime prevention and crime responsive schemes, but social policies to correct inequity must be also be present.

Real victims

Victims have conventionally not figured centrally (if at all) in criminological research and crime policy making. However, by the end of the twentieth century, victims moved from the margins of the criminological agenda to be key players (Zedner, 1997). That is, the profile of the victim has been raised in criminology theory and research, as well as in the political domain. In Britain, schemes have been introduced to incorporate 'impact statements' by victims within the evidence collected by the Crown Prosecution Service, and pressure groups representing special classifications of victim have been set up. For example, 'Mothers Against Murder and Aggression' gives support to, and campaigns on behalf of, relatives who have lost loved ones as a consequence of such massacres as that which occurred in Dunblane. In the USA, 'Families of Murder Victims' was set up to provide support and advocacy, lobby the media and policy makers, and introduce 'antiviolence' education programmes into schools and colleges.

The impact of crime on the life of individuals and the community is common and wide-ranging. Reviewing both quantitative and qualitative research, Lucia Zedner (1997) records that short-term psychological effects (for example, fear, anxiety, guilt, a feeling of loss, depression, disturbed sleeping and eating patterns, and a sense of having had one's life intruded upon) occur for the victim following most types of crime. Where physical and/or sexual assault has taken place, these symptoms can last for years and are more severe. The more socially isolated the victim is, the more intense the aftermath.

These effects have become categorized as 'post-traumatic stress disorder', a medical syndrome that can be viewed as a specific outcome of crime-ridden Western societies. Moreover, the repercussions of crime for the associates of the victim (described as 'secondary victims', 'indirect victims' or 'co-victims') are now being understood. This is of particular importance in cases of murder where not only the relatives and friends of the victim are affected, but also those who were present at the murder – even if they did not know the victim – may suffer psychological damage:

> The wider impact of crime on secondary or 'indirect' victims is increasingly recognised in the literature. The most obvious example is that of the families of murder victims ... Although they are not primary victims they suffer perhaps the most profound trauma of any crime victim. The trauma of sudden bereavement is often compounded by the viciousness of the attack or the senselessness of the killing. For those who witness homicide or other non-fatal assaults, feelings of shock or guilt for failing to intervene may be profound, and onlookers too may be victims. (Zedner, 1997, p593)

For the nearest relative of someone murdered, the anguish is immediate and profound. Not only will the secondary victim be psychologically traumatized by the murder, but subsequent events will also heighten the experience of loss. He or she will in all likelihood have to identify the body, sort out the financial affairs of the victim, make the funeral arrangements, be interviewed by the police (and assessed as a potential suspect) and possibly have to deal with the media. All of these responsibilities, whilst perhaps having a ritualistic and therefore, to a limited degree, 'desensitising' side-effect, add tangible realities to the sense of privation.

Deborah Spungen (1998), whose own daughter was murdered at the age of 20 years, vividly describes the feeling of devastation on the news that a loved one has been 'unlawfully killed':

> the blackest hell accompanied by a pain so intense that even breathing becomes an unendurable labor. (Spungen, 1998, pXIX)

However, as Spungen explains, beyond the instantaneous emotional turmoil, the distress that accompanies the bureaucratic procedures surrounding modern death, and the reactivation of these emotions during the trial, there quite conceivably lies a lifetime of fury and grief. Moreover, Spungen records that the secondary victim can undergo an illogical sense of guilt about the murder, which may be contributed to by the reactions of others. That is, a not-infrequent response from associates of the victim, which may be implied rather than stated openly, is to hold the secondary victim in some way or another culpable.

The major contribution of NLR to formal criminological theory has indeed been to draw attention to the role – and suffering – of the victim. Although by no means the first theoretical perspective to focus on 'victimology', NLR has been successful in providing a rationale for the victim's inclusion within criminological theorizing.

A number of points can be made about the role played by victims. First, victims are not merely randomly selected by their tormentors. As has been discussed in Chapter 3, many victims of homicide (and other types of violent crime) have strong personal connections to the offender, and a significant subsection of those who fall prey to one form of crime will succumb to others. Second, not only do victims play a crucial part in defining whether or not an 'incident' becomes classified as a 'crime' (for example, by deciding to inform the police in the first place and by formally identifying the culprit), but also those who suffer from the actions of criminals may themselves become vituperators at some stage. That is, in some situations, the line between victim and culprit is overstepped – for example, the sexually abused may become paedophiles, drug addicts may become drug pushers, or a householder who is being burgled may 'over-react' and be prosecuted for 'violence against the person'.

Furthermore, the phenomenon of 'repeat victimization', whereby psychosocial elements in the behaviour and circumstances of 'victims' may contribute to their own predicament, has been used by the government and the police in their bid to reduce the crime rate. In a number of pilot studies, repeat victims of burglary have been supplied with crime prevention paraphernalia (locks, bolts and alarms) and advice. This goes hand-in-hand with the police concentrating their efforts on prolific offenders (that is, those who are known to commit a disproportionate number of offences). In one town in Britain, this approach has seen a reduction in domestic burglary of 21% (Home Office, 1998c).

NLR theorists produced the idea of 'the square of crime' in their analysis of criminality. For Young & Mathew (1992), the problem of crime is denoted as the complex interaction and relationship between four key elements (which make up the square of crime): the agencies of social control (primarily the police and the judiciary), the public, the offender and the victim. All of these elements, argue the realists, have to be considered both in the production of policies on crime at national and local levels, and in the handling of particular crimes.

In Britain, victims of crime receive automatic help (in the form of information leaflets and/or counselling) from a national charity, 'Victim Support'. This charity functions independently but is part-funded by the government. More vitally, however, the 'victim perspective' is included formally in the criminal justice system of Britain, Australia, New Zealand, North America and other parts of Europe. Under the banner of 'restorative justice', the police and the courts now recognize that crime is detrimental to those who fall prey to the criminal in ways other than the obvious loss of possessions and/or physical injury, as well as to society in general. This staggering insight has indeed led to the promotion of a 'balanced' way of dealing with the offender, which involves the victim and community representatives, as well the state. The following extract from an information leaflet produced by the British Thames Valley police force sets the case for the restorative approach and indicates its priorities:

> Restorative justice deals with the impact of crime and criminal behaviour on our communities in an effective way. Its primary aim is to repair harm and resolve the underlying causes of inappropriate behaviour. This is achieved by restoring the parties affected by such behaviour, rather than the traditional approach of seeking to punish and blame offenders ... Central to restorative justice is the balanced approach; providing opportunities for victims, communities and offenders with a stake in an incident to contribute to the justice process. It recognises that crime violates people and communities not just the State, weakens relationships and harms community safety.
> (Thames Valley Police, 1997, p5)

Moreover, the British government has published a victim's 'charter'. In this document, standards of service by the various criminal agencies are laid out, and information about, for example, being a prosecution witness, court procedures and compensation is provided. Reassuringly, the charter also explains to the victim that the police 'will do their best to catch the person responsible for your crime', and sensitively, where a relative has suffered from a serious crime or has been killed, the guardians of law and order will 'give you the relevant information pack to help you' (Home Office, 1996, p2).

The principles of restorative justice also have an application to the way in which the mentally disordered are dealt with in society. For example, I argue that when community or institutional care initiatives are planned, the public at a local level should be consulted – in order to inform and therefore disarm the potential volatile reaction that local communities are likely to have when not made familiar with any new provision (Morrall, 1999b).

Despite its acceptance of the effect of 'relative deprivation' in the production of crime, NLR has aimed to steer a middle course through the political agendas of both the left and the right:

> NLR wishes to avoid the worst excesses of both the 'right' and 'left' idealist approaches to the problem of crime in Britain. The right is accused of over-dramatising the problem, whilst the left has minimalised the crime issue as merely a form of ideological mystification on behalf of the capitalist state.
> (Hughes, 1991, p18)

Notwithstanding this attempt by the sponsors of NLR to hit the middle ground politically (that is, by arguing for a structurally modi-fied 'liberal democracy'), it is, however, probable that those on the left have been offended. This is not only because the criminal has been upstaged by the victim (and the left like nothing more than to defend those whom they perceive to be casualties of the capitalist system), but particularly also because 'better policing' has been proposed as a way forward in the management of crime.

In what can be seen as in one sense undermining the victimol-ogy movement, Michael Gottfredson and Travis Hirschi (1990) have argued that most criminology theories ignore the traits of criminal acts. They point out that most crime (whether 'organized, 'blue' or 'white' collar) is trivial, mundane, opportunistic, requiring little specialist skill or knowledge to carry out, and highly predictable in terms of where and when it occurs. Repeating ideas originally used in classical theory (see Chapter 4), they claim that 'impulsiveness' and low self-control are the standard constituents of criminal behav-iour. Criminals by and large aim at the immediate gratification of their needs, without much 'rational' attention to either how their actions affect others or the long-term consequences to themselves. Behavioural patterns that lead to crime are indoctrinated in child-hood because of parental inadequacies (for example, a lack of super-vision, oppressive and/or irregular discipline and rejection) and are inclined to be lifelong.

Consequently, for Gottfredson & Hirschi, neither the school nor peer association is responsible for delinquency. There is, therefore, a rejection of the proposition put forward by Sutherland (1947) that the positive labelling experienced by young delinquents as members of countercultural gangs ('crime is its own reward') transcends the negative reaction of the community to their behaviour. Moreover, for Gottfredson & Hirschi, criminality is not caused by such social conditions as unemployment.

So, if criminality is not dependent on, and reinforced by, social disadvantage, poor educational experiences and peer association, then, as Brannigan (1997) notes, attempts to address the behaviour of the individual through individual 'restorative' training may be successful. However, an extrapolation from this position is that a victim-centred criminal justice system based on employment-based rehabilitation programmes or shaming offenders in the audience of their victims is unlikely to be effective.

There is, of course, a major fault with projecting the view that parental inadequacies cause juvenile crime without exploring the connection between patterns of socialization and social structures. Robert Sampson and John Laub (1993) used the secondary analysis of a huge data set from a study compiled by Sheldon and Eleanor Glueck (1950, 1968) over a period of 25 years in which the lives of hundreds of delinquent and non-delinquent boys were examined. What Sampson & Laub were able to identify was that social and economic marginalization creates the circumstances in which failure at the level of primary socialization is probable. This again, therefore, may lead to the conclusion that the confrontation of criminals with the material and emotional consequences of their acts will, in the long term at any rate, have little effect.

Lucia Zedner provides a warning concerning the success of the victimology movement:

> The danger is that concern for the victim may be used to justify the pursuit of punitivism in their name and the promotion of victim's interests over those of the offender. (Zedner, 1997, p607)

However, in the case of mentally disordered people committing violent acts, the introduction of the victim perspective does not rest on challenging the perpetrator, clearly (in the main) an inhuman and counterproductive tactic. What needs to be accepted as routine in the development of national and local policies is the concept of 'victim' in its broader sense. This includes the notion of 'community as victim' and the realization that the scenario of murder is multilayered – and more so when the offender is mentally disordered as he or she is also a victim.

Realistically mad

My proposition is that realism can be applied profitably to the understanding of madness in society. A realist account of madness implies that while there are difficulties in extending Western-centric psychiatric disease categories and concepts universally, this does not deny the 'lived reality' of mental disorder for both the sufferer and his or her associates.

In a discussion on the nature of schizophrenia in cultures other than the West, Paul Hirst and Penny Woolley observe that the occurrence of substantial variations in incidence and forms of mental disorder across the world does not necessarily imply that madness as such is an invention. They conclude:

> We cannot dispense with the category of 'schizophrenia' – clinical observation is not an illusion. Nor can we dispense with analytical concepts, but we must be prepared to limit and modify them in conditions of application other than their own institutional and discursive sites. (Hirst & Woolley, 1982, p115)

Crime and mental disorder may have different cultural and historical representations, but the act of separating what each society determines as 'normal' from what is held to be 'deviant' is a constant. A society will invariably condemn and control those behaviours (and thoughts) which do not fit into the predominant mode of conduct for that society.

Moreover, what in the industrialized world became described as 'schizophrenia', 'manic depressive psychosis' or 'psychopathy' has its equivalent in each and every other culture. The transitive knowledge object of insanity presents as a culturally distinct 'condition', but there is an intransitive knowledge foundation to all abnormalities of mind.

The application of realist principles to mental disorder is of particular relevance at a time when both public fears about risk, and a collapse in the credibility of professional practice, have pushed the state into rethinking its policies and laws. Realism, put to use in the analysis of homicides by mentally disordered people, allows for the inclusion of all relevant constituents: the necessary implementation of social control functions by the state and its agencies of social control; genuine public anxiety; the predicament of the mentally disordered in hospitals, prisons and the community; and the psychological, social and financial needs of victims.

A realist perspective implies that there is a 'real' basis to the incidents of homicide committed by the mentally disordered. Realism challenges the belief, expressed by so many members of the psychiatric establishment, that murders by the mentally disordered are inescapable facts of life, and that potential or actual killers are not amenable to treatment. That is, realism betrays impossibilism.

Summary

Realist theory is an integrative paradigm that has prospered from the deficiencies in both positivist and constructionist attempts to explain crime and deviancy. It has the merit of not only respecting insuperable realities about, for example, the male physique and hormones in the generation of crime, and the part played by social conditions, but also submitting a comprehensive model to help to relieve 'the problem of crime'. Most importantly, realism has given the victim a say in criminological theorising and policy making.

Realism applied to Madness and Murder leads to the following propositions. First, madness has a reality for both the sufferers and their families – it exists to all intents and purposes. Second, some mentally disordered 'folk devils' are dangerous, and a minority do commit homicide (although many more kill themselves). Third, these acts of homicide are not the consequence of labelling or moral panic, nor, as postmodern conjecture might imply, are they a 'lifestyle choice'. Fourth, any homicide by a mentally disordered person is a social calamity that creates a host of casualties – the victim and his or her family, the perpetrator and the community. Fifth, society and the mentally disordered need protecting. These propositions will be examined further in Chapter 8.

Chapter 8
The terror

In the preceding chapter, a realist paradigm was proffered as the most credible approach to understanding criminality and deviance. The argument was made that crime and deviance are indeed shaped by social factors (as well as some biological stimuli). Realists, therefore, want to transform the structures in society that make antisocial behaviour more probable; but realists also testify that crime and deviance have a detrimental impact on law-abiding citizens and society, and should, therefore, be combated even before any structural changes come to pass.

Applying realism to mental disorder, I argue in this chapter that the fear from 'mad murderers' throughout the 1990s in Britain was 'real' in the sense that a significant number of people were killed. Moreover, I suggest that it was in part the 'defensive' reaction of the psychiatric disciplines of medicine and nursing that fuelled a 'media panic' about the mad.

What I am engaging in here, however, is not a disputation about statistics. Whether there are 500, 50 or five 'mad murders' annually is not the focus of my thesis. It is the repercussions of murders by the mentally disordered on a multitude of lives and on social perceptions (warranted or otherwise) that is my concern. I begin this chapter, therefore, with a review of the debate about the media's role in creating terror with regard to the mentally disordered living in the community. This is followed by a presentation of the research design and results from my own five-year study of the media's coverage of 'mad murders'.

Media hype

Mental disorder is hardly ever out of the news in Britain. There are thousands of stories each year in the media and academic articles about, for example, community provision (or the lack of it), abuse in institutions, genetic and pharmaceutical research, stigma and intolerance, and enterprising initiatives from the DoH.

Media coverage of mental health issues is only part of a complex set of interrelated factors working to formulate public perceptions about 'madness' (Pilgrim & Rogers, 1999). It is, therefore, extremely difficult to measure accurately the extent to which the media strengthens, adjusts or manufactures public opinion towards the mentally disordered.

It would seem, however, that while studies since the 1950s into public attitudes have identified the media's role in reinforcing a traditional image of the mentally disordered as unpredictable and potentially violent (Colombo, 1997), there is not necessarily any consistency within the public's collective conscience. For example, Wolff et al. (1996a, 1996b) conducted a survey of community attitudes towards, and knowledge about, the mentally disordered in specific London districts. They discovered that the socio-demographic characteristics of local communities were important determinants. Whilst only a minority of the respondents in their study (9%) objected to having neighbours who were 'ex-psychiatric patients', those in higher social classes were more tolerant. Furthermore, respondents living in households with children had an increased level of fear with regard to mentally disordered people living in their vicinity, and a greater expression of the need to 'control' through hospitalization existed amongst certain ethnic minority groups (Asians, Afro-Caribbeans and Africans). Wolff et al. attribute much of the negativity they discovered in their study to a deficiency in education about the mentally disordered.

Moreover, data from studies of public attitudes towards mentally disordered people are used for competing political agendas. For example, Wolff and his co-researchers are in favour of interventions that increase the acceptance of community-based mental health services:

As negative attitudes are associated with lack of knowledge, education may
possibly improve attitudes and help patients' reintegration into the community. (Wolff et al., 1996b, p196)

This is in marked contrast to the conclusions drawn by Michael
Howlett (1998), Director of the Zito Trust, in a study of the effects on
the homicidal behaviour of the mentally disordered of not taking
prescribed medication. A registered charity, the Zito Trust was set up
in 1994 following the death of Jonathan Zito (see below) in order to
lobby parliament for changes to the policy of care in the community,
which it considers has serious deficiencies, particularly with regard
to the needs of the severely mentally disordered.

Howlett analysed data from a 1997 MORI national survey of
attitudes towards the mentally disordered and mental health services
(which contained a representative sample of 1804 respondents). He
argues that media focus on homicide and violence by mentally disordered offenders does not increase stigmatization. He observes that,
at the same time as speculation about the dangerousness of the
mentally disordered had been rife in the media, 72% of the respondents in the MORI poll believed that, with adequate support and
treatment, people with schizophrenia could live successfully in the
community.

Nor is there a standard presentation of 'mad' imagery across the
various sections of the media. The visual and motion-based docu-
mentation of social events in television programmes has an effect
different from that of the static and largely textual chronicling of
newspapers and magazines. Moreover, both 'positive' and 'negative'
imagery may appear on television within one evening's viewing or in
the same edition of a newspaper.

However, although ambiguity abounds with respect to research
into public perceptions and the effect of the media, there is a virtually universal and historically unprecedented level of unanimity
amongst and between the psychiatric disciplines about the danger
being posed by the mentally disordered living in the community and
the role of the media. For example, psychiatrists Professor Pamela
Taylor and Professor John Gunn, from the Institute of Psychiatry in
London, argue that a 'popular delusion' exists about the threat posed
by mentally disorderd people (Taylor & Gunn, 1999). This prohibits
what they describe as 'moderate and scientific steps' being imple-

mented to determine and solve the needs of those with serious psychiatric problems, and to resolve any backlash from caring for this group of people within the community. Taylor & Gunn are in no doubt as to who is responsible for nurturing this 'misunderstanding' about the risk posed by the mentally disordered:

> Fed by highly selected information in the mass media about their [that is, mentally disordered people's] very rare contribution to one type of tragedy – homicide – the public and politicians believe through the mass media, that unless people with a mental disorder are once more segregated, the streets will not be safe. (Taylor & Gunn, 1999, p9)

Responding to the move from liberal to post-liberal government approaches to care of the mentally disordered, Taylor & Gunn argue that it makes no sense to reformulate mental health policy on the basis of the (murderous) behaviour of a few people. Calculating that up to a thousand people annually die at the hands of 'normal' murderers and dangerous drivers, and a further 3500–4000 people die in accidents on the road, the public, they observe, are at far greater risk of being killed by those who are ostensibly sane. Therefore, although there is a 'small but important' problem of homicide committed by the mentally disordered, incarcerating all mentally disordered people 'to save 40 or so lives' is comparable to the proscription of private motoring (Taylor & Gunn, 1999, p10).

Taylor & Gunn use the analogy of winning the jackpot in the National Lottery, arguing that the odds of doing so are similar to those of being killed by someone who is mentally disordered. They underscore the illogicality, as they see it, of public alarm (which has resulted in the re-establishment of asylum care) by pointing out that the victim is usually a parent, sibling, offspring, spouse or some other person close to the mad murderer.

Despite the overall tenor of Taylor & Gunn's position, they (reassuringly) recognize that, however small the threat by mentally disordered people, there is an obligation on the psychiatric disciplines to reduce the risk. Moreover, they admit that they may have a role in refuting what they consider to be 'myths' about the mentally disordered:

> Psychiatrists may help themselves, their services and their patients by taking an information-based but higher profile in public and political debate to

counter popular and stigmatising mythologies about people with mental
disorder. (Taylor & Gunn, 1999, p14)

In 1997, the Health Education Authority (HEA) conducted a
study of newspaper reports that had made reference to mental disorder
during the previous year. MIND, the mental health charity, supplied
over 1000 press cuttings from 19 daily and Sunday British newspapers
(both broad-sheet and tabloid) for the study. These were then evaluated
for frequency and signification using the 'Impact Media Analysis
Service'. The key findings from the study are that: there was a clear
connection of mental disorder to crime and violence (self-injury and
the injury of others) in 46% of the stories; over 40% of the stories
contained pejorative words and phrases about mental disorder and
mentally disordered people (for example, 'bonkers'); and more than
20% of the coverage provided explicitly 'positive' messages about the
capability of sufferers to lead worthwhile lives and the treatability of
mental disorder.

Overall, the promulgation in the 'highbrow' (that is, broad-sheet)
and 'gutter' (that is, tabloid) press of 'negative' imagery was remarkably
comparable – 67% and 75% respectively. However, although broad-
sheet coverage accounted for most of the stories (80%), the HEA found
that it was the tabloids that were responsible for most of the prejudicial
portrayal of mental disorder. Moreover, because of their far higher
readership, the tabloids deliver their interpretation of mental disorder
more widely. For example, when Brazil lost to France in the final of the
1998 World Cup soccer tournament, one of the Brazilian players
(Ronaldo Luiz Nazario da Lima) was targeted the following day (14th
July) by the press for his perceived failure to live up to expectations.
With a hugely increased audience as a result of the popularity of the
World Cup event, a British tabloid newspaper (the *Daily Mirror*) ran
with the following headline emblazoned across its front page:

BRAZIL NUTTER: Ronaldo had mental breakdown night before France
final

There is also a tendency amongst the tabloids to produce far
more extensive features on a particular incident. For example, in
1998, one case of homicide by a man purported to be mentally
disordered attracted in one issue: 5 pages in the *Daily Express*, 8 in the
Daily Mail, 9 in the *Daily Mirror* and 11 in the *Sun*.

The reporting of a man who had approached the late Princess Diana, when she was talking to bystanders on a visit to Liverpool, in another tabloid newspaper takes some beating with respect to the negative presentation of mental disorder. The *Daily Star* (9th November, 1995) printed a five-page story on the man, concentrating on his 'mad' behaviour and admission to psychiatric institutions. Phrases such as 'the devil's son', 'nutter's kids are afraid of him' and 'ex-girlfriend said ... he could have killed her' were preceded by the headline:

> HE'S A RAVING NUTTER: World exclusive on Mental patient who stole a kiss from Di

But, as Mathew Engel (1996) observes, writing in the *Guardian*, the traditional splitting of the UK press on the basis of 'taste' and 'quality' has been undermined through increased competition. In the 1990s, the advent of new broad-sheet newspapers (for example, the *Independent*), the drastic lowering of the price of others (for example, *The Times*), and a rapidly enlarging range of media choice for news reports, forced the remaining broad-sheets to rethink their marketing strategy. As if to underline the extent to which the *Guardian* (a broad-sheet) has mutated, alongside Engel's article is a naked picture of the British actress, Helen Mirren. The accompanying text (written in a tongue-in-cheek style) mentions her age as 50 years, and refers to her appearance thus:

> Blonde locks curling onto naked shoulders, soft flesh, her hand provocatively flung across her bare chest...

In Australia, where a similar process has occurred, one quality newspaper (the *Advertiser*, based in Adelaide) crossed the traditional divide by changing its format from broad-sheet to tabloid in 1997. Many of the UK broad-sheets developed compact sections embellished with the type of lurid and/or salacious captions and articles previously only seen in the tabloids. For example, an article about a relationship between two members of the House of Lords (former Chief Whip Baroness Llewelyn-Davies and former deputy Speaker Lord Alport) appeared in the tabloid portion of the *Guardian* (8 March 1999) with the following headline:

LOVE ACROSS THE WOOLSACK

Although it could be argued that journalists from the broad-sheets are frequently employing irony by borrowing the tabloid style (as with the Helen Mirren example above), McRobbie & Thornton (1995) observe that this does not provide absolution from the effects of such headlines. Paradoxically, whereas there is considerable suspicion amongst readers of the most popular (in terms of sales) tabloids, such as the *Sun*, about the accuracy of stories (Pursehouse, 1991), the 'mocking' formula that newspapers such as the *Guardian* use may not be always be appreciated. For example, the linguisti-cally and intellectually resourceful journalist Joanna Coles created the following title in the *Guardian* (28 September 1996) about the sacking of presenter Paul Gambaccini from BBC's Radio 3 and his subsequent reaction to the criticism from its audience that had led to his removal:

MAD AXED MAN HITS BACK AT RADIO 3

In his critique of the Welsh National Opera's production of Benjamin Britten's *Peter Grimes*, a story based in an east of England fishing village about the cruelty of the eponymous Grimes, Andrew Clements, writing in the *Guardian* (18 February 1999) came up with the caption:

A PSYCHOTIC ON THE LOOSE IN SUFFOLK

These reformulations of the recurrent and stereotypical 'mad axeman' and 'violent nutters in the community' headlines are inge-nious. However, they are also inflammatory and liable to misinter-pretation if the accompanying narrative is not read and its paradoxical intent recognized.

Furthermore, broad-sheet newspapers at times 'dress up' stories and incidents in what is purported to be sincere critique. However, despite the interweaving of 'facts' and 'expert opinion', they may not have any greater merit than the equivalent found in the more blatant (and perhaps more candid) 'gutter press'.

For example, in the same edition of the *Guardian* as the 'wool-sack' story, a picture taken from the contentious film *Crash* made an appearance. The film, by director David Cronenberg, is an adaptation of a novel about a couple who seek sexual gratification from their involvement in car collisions. In the picture used by the *Guardian*, the emergency services are attending to what appears to be an horrific accident involving a number of vehicles. Alongside this graphic scene are photographs of a number of celebrities who have died in car crashes – Albert Camus, Grace Kelly, James Dean, Marc Bolan, Jayne Mansfield and Jackson Pollock. Within the body of the article are the results of an Australian research study that recorded incidents of people having sexual fantasies prior to crashing their cars. There is also a commentary by a representative of the UK-based Royal Automobile Club on sexual frustration causing irritability whilst driving.

On the same page, but in a separate article, an interview with television actress Rebecca Lacey is transcribed, ending with the question 'Have you ever had sex in a car?' The reply from Lacey, above a picture of her leaning against a car with the inscription 'Racey Lacey with her Toyota', is 'No I haven't. So there's something to look forward to.'

The implication from the HEA study discussed above is that the press coverage continues to pursue a deprecatory stance with regard to the mentally disordered. However, the HEA admits that the degree to which this is done is less than that found in previous studies, and that:

> Many of the articles examined gave a balanced and well-informed coverage.
> The landscape of mental ill health pictured in the national press is not just
> one of axe-wielding psychos, but can be a more welcoming place, peopled
> by men and women experiencing a range of problems which can, poten-
> tially, affect anyone. (Health Education Authority, 1997, p2)

Such research tends to accept the position that the media 'shapes' public opinion.

As has been discussed in Chapter 6, there is an undeniable refining of reality as a consequence of either unpremeditated or deliberate editorial decisions about which story to use and how to present narrative and pictures. But the notion that the audience is merely a passive recipient of manipulated messages adheres to a crude form of social determinism:

the general public should be given more credit for its ability to transcend sensationalist newspaper reporting, absorb evidence, reflect upon it, and then form a balanced and coherent view. (Howlett, 1998, p87)

Shulmit Ramon, Professor of inter-professional health and social studies at Anglia Polytechnic University in the UK, reports on her research into British newspapers and British and Italian television documentaries (Ramon, 1996). Ramon argues for the adoption of a Marxist discourse analytical framework for the study of the media's approach to mental disorder. This framework, Ramon suggests, will demystify the meaning and context of media coverage, and challenge what she considers to be 'major distortions by the people who manufacture the news' (Ramon, 1996, p196).

However, Ramon's *mélange* of Marxist and (postmodern) discourse precepts produces an inconsistent collage of analytical propositions. For example, the Marxist assertion that the media is involved in the production of 'myth' and 'distortion' implies that there is some 'reality' (or at least a preferential world-view) to be discovered once the mystifying and hegemonic effects of capitalism ideology are removed. An axiom of postmodernist theorizing, however, is ideological fragmentation and absolute relativism – no one belief system or reality can be more veracious than another.

Psychiatric implacability

I do not automatically accept this antagonistic view of the role and effect of the media. In embracing a realist perspective, I appreciate that all media stories need to be understood in terms of their preconceptualizations and moulding of 'facts', but I reject the proposition that the media exists in, and fosters, a 'hyper-real' domain.

Furthermore, receiving the 'gaze' of the media and the public may not only result in negative depictions of mentally disordered people. Andrew Sims, Professor of psychiatry at St James's University Hospital, Leeds, and former President of the Royal College of Psychiatrists, refers to the widespread media interest over the case in 1993 of Ben Silcock. Silcock, diagnosed as suffering from schizophrenia, had been badly mauled after climbing into a lion's den at London Zoo. Sims records that the Silcock incident led to a year in which mental disorder was constantly in the public arena. Sims attributes this in part to the fact that Silcock's father was a journalist. However, Sims reflects on both the positive and negative effects of media and public curiosity and apprehension about the bizarre and visible behaviour of the psychotic:

> Turning the spotlight upon psychiatry has good and bad consequences. For instance, it draws attention to both the need for more resources and also to the inadequacies of the present service and, by inference, the providers of that service. It draws attention both to the possibility of and the need for psychiatric treatment, and also its failures. It draws attention both to the difficulty of the job of psychiatrists and also to their occasional incompetence. It draws attention to both the vulnerability of psychiatric patients, and their potential dangerousness. (Sims, 1996, p86)

Mike Hazelton (1996) examined 'media discourse' relating to mental health in two Australian newspapers (*The Examiner* and *The Australian*). Hazelton takes the well-rehearsed 'cultural studies' position (of, for example, Lupton, 1992) that the media is responsible for setting the parameters within which what counts as news, and what can be legitimately debated politically, is predetermined. Hazelton reports that the news stories covered in his study (for one year – 1994), dealing with a range of divergent themes, included: (a) accounts of bizarre behaviour, such as the mentally disordered Indonesian man who had to undergo surgery to remove cutlery he had swallowed; (b) glorified descriptions of medical-scientific achievements, particularly with reference to psycho-pharmaceuticals; (c) 'moral tales' about the lifestyles of public figures (including psychiatrists) leading to madness or self-destruction, and the disintegration of social norms bringing about high levels of suicide amongst the young; and (d) the use of lay remedies (for example, massage, music or drinking tea) in dealing with the stress of everyday living.

Hazelton, however, claims to have identified an 'underlying ideological unity' in his study. He states that 'disorder', 'crisis' and 'risk' are predominant elements in the news stories. These elements are contained in discussions that focus on the danger to the public following the deinstitutionalization of the mentally disordered and the mismanagement of the policy of community care by the mental health disciplines. For Hazelton, the concentration on these elements in the context of the division in mental health policy between asylum and community care emerges from the 'predictable narratives' and 'preferred images' held by the press.

Indeed, the Australian press would appear to have sustained the same 'framing strategy' that Hazelton believes he has detected. For example, an Adelaide newspaper in 1997 (three years after Hazelton collected his data), in an extensive article by journalist Fiona Clark on the (dis)organization of local mental health services, used the headline 'Out of Control'. The text of the article chronicles details from the report of the State Coroner into a number of murders by and suicides of people who had been diagnosed as schizophrenic:

> On December 3, 1992, David Tzeegankoff walked out of his doctor's office ... Tzeegankoff, frustrated at the progress of his psychiatric treatment, had stabbed and bashed her [his doctor] to death. The following year, Geoffrey Hogarth bashed his own mother to death with a rock and the year after that, Frank Ciampi slit his mother's throat. Then within months of each other in 1994 three men suicided by lying down on railway tracks in the path of an oncoming train ... This week, the State Coroner linked all six of the deaths in a damning finding on the State's [South Australia's] mental health system. Barely a corner of the system remained untouched, with the coroner ... criticising everything from the facilities to the treatment itself. (Clark, 1997)

Hazelton understands that the media prioritizes issues that are already of major public interest. That is, whilst arguing on the one hand that agendas are set by the media, he accepts that those issues (such as mental health) which have prominence within the public domain are also given prominence in news reports. Furthermore, Hazelton embraces the critique of the media by Hall and his colleagues (Hall et al., 1978) that there is a process of 'making sense' of events in the production of news items. In doing so, however, there is the potential to sanction or stigmatize certain groups, and embellish or trivialize particular incidents.

The media frequently uses published accounts from independent inquiries, coroners' reports or governmental papers. That is, although there is 'overemphasis', 'selection' and 'reframing', there is no discernible falsification of events on any major scale. The story by Clark of patients who later killed themselves and of others receiving inadequate medication at the hands of ill-trained medical practitioners is only 'made up' in the sense of its being a 'textual reconstruction' of reality – and not an invention.

In all cases of homicide perpetrated by the mentally disordered (defined as people who have been in contact with the specialist psychiatric services) in England and Wales, an independent inquiry must be instituted. This requirement, suggests Matt Muijen (1996), a psychiatrist and Director of the Sainsbury Centre for Mental Health in London, has led to an 'inquiry culture'. In this culture, the actions of mental health staff come under intense, and thereby, for Muijen, unfair, scrutiny from 'cynical' panels. Nigel Eastman (referred to in Hall, 1996), head of forensic psychiatry at St George's Hospital Medical School in London, believes that a mandatory inquiry system is particularly unfair to medical staff. For Eastman, a potentially unjust treatment of doctors results from the way in which the inquiries connect cause to culpability. That is, not only do the members of the inquiry panel attempt to find out what circumstances led to a killing, but they also seek to attach blame.

Moreover, it has been argued cogently that such an arrangement results in an undue focus on homicides committed by the mentally disordered compared with 'normal' murderers (Peay, 1996). This has the consequence of amplifying further the social disapproval for this form of deviancy. The Royal College of Psychiatrists (1997) claims that not only is the inquiry system too expensive and deleterious for staff morale, but it has also damaged public confidence in the mental health service. Furthermore, psychiatrists Taylor & Gunn (1999) go as far as to infer that lobby groups such as the Zito Trust, set up to influence mental health policy following the killing of Jane Zito's husband by Christopher Clunis, have inadvertently led to more control over the mentally disordered than is warranted. Christopher Clunis, diagnosed as a paranoid schizophrenic, stabbed to death 27-year-old Jonathan Zito at Finsbury Park underground train station, London, in 1992. Clunis was convicted of manslaughter and ordered to be detained indefinitely.

Chris Heginbotham, Chief Executive of East and North Hertfordshire Health Authority and ex-Director of MIND, blames 'lurid media coverage of crimes by mentally ill people' for encouraging a perception of the mad as dangerous (Heginbotham, 1998, p1052). Muijen (1996) traces the beginning of the association of the mentally disordered living in the community with danger to an incident in 1984. In July of that year, social worker Isabel Schwarz was killed by her former client Sharon Campbell, who had a history of violent attacks. The findings of the inquiry into the killing of Isabel Schwarz highlighted poor communication between mental health staff (particularly with regard to Campbell's previous assaults), a situation routinely found in the mental health arena. For Muijen, it was the Campbell case that set the agenda for eventual changes in mental health policy that meant that health, social and voluntary agencies had to prepare 'care programmes' for discharged patients, and for the formal registering of 'designated' patients living in the community.

According to Muijen, other 'dramatic events' in the early 1990s, such as Ben Silcock being found in the lion's den, and the death of Jonathan Zito at the hands of Christopher Clunis, produced a 'moral panic' and thereby a refocusing of policy. He argues that the attention of the media on the seemingly unpredictable behaviour of mentally disordered people resulted in the government defaulting on a long-standing pledge to support community care. That is, for Muijen, rather than attempting to correct the faults in community care, the government capitulated in the face of public demands for greater protection. The DoH, observes Muijen, decided to address defective coordination amongst the mental health disciplines and to create more secure accommodation. However, it did not at the time invest in measures that would potentially have corrected the deficiencies in community care, such as intensive outreach teams and a restructuring of the work of community psychiatric nursing. The latter, insists Muijen, would have meant the government would have had to allocate extra resources to mental health.

It is, of course, a mistake to argue that pulling away from the policy of community care does not have resource implications. For example, the building of a new secure unit costs as much as £9 million (Department of Health, 1998f). Moreover, in its declared intention to modernize the mental health system of care, the British government in 1998 assigned an additional £700 million – over a period of three years – to the funding of mental health services (Department of Health, 1998g).

Muijen, perhaps inadvertently (given his support for the argument that the 'failure' of community care has been brought about by underfunding rather than being wrong in principle), draws attention to the counterproductive consequences of a defensive stance by the psychiatric disciplines:

> The publicity around reports [of inquiries into killings by the mentally
> disordered] has created a sense of random and irrational danger. *The
> public are angered by the message that it is not the fault of vulnerable patients, who are
> victims too, but of an inadequate system.* (Muijen, 1996, p149, emphasis
> added)

That is, Muijen appears to realize that by avoiding the responsibility
for major shortcomings in practice, and for claiming persistently that
it is media hype (and largely a problem of resources), mental health
professionals have promulgated public unease.

The public has not accepted that any threat posed by the
mentally disordered living within their midst is either non-existent or
negligible. No matter what the justification for claiming that the
press has merely embarked on one of its regular and self-serving
outbursts of moral indignation, mental health practitioners have
themselves hindered the cause of community care by not only being
seen to be inefficient but, in an unprecedented spectacle of professional hubris, also castigating the victims (i.e. the families of those
who have been killed and the community as a whole) for indulging in
the 'delusion' that the mentally disordered are dangerous.

On the other hand, the British government did not hesitate to
take a patronizing view of the capacity of the citizen to judge what is
and what is not a bona fide threat to his or her safety. Nor did it
refrain from attacking the media's overzealous desire to connect
madness to murder, or from questioning the dependability of the
mental health disciplines:

> Whilst adverse media reporting can distort the relationship between mental
> illness and homicide, the public have the right to be concerned ... Typically,
> there is poor communication and co-ordination between professionals and
> agencies, and a failure to listen to warning signs from relatives, carers and
> others. (Department of Health, 1998g, p14)

For Ray Rowden, psychiatric nurse, former Chief Executive of
the Security Psychiatric Services Commissioning Board and *clerici
vagantes*, it would seem that a policy that has at its centre the welfare
of the public is to be unequivocally rejected:

> it would appear that the starting point of public policy for the mentally-ill
> must be protection of the public. Safety, it seems, is to be top of the policy
> pops. This approach is wrong. (Rowden, 1998)

Rowden admits that the mental health disciplines may have what he describes as a 'secondary role' in reassuring the public, but he offers the *gratis dictum* that their primary task is to provide 'those living with mental illness with good diagnosis, treatment rehabilitation and care'. By not accepting that psychiatric medicine and nursing have a dual responsibility to safeguard the mentally disordered (as well as provide treatment) and protect the public, it is my contention that the fear of killers living in the community is exacerbated and public tolerance exasperated.

A well-documented exhibition of defensiveness by psychiatrists occurred after the conviction in England of Michael Stone in 1998 for the killing of a woman and her daughter. At the trial, Stone was described as having been treated within the psychiatric system for a severe personality disorder. There was an ensuing clash in the media between the Home Secretary (Jack Straw) and the president of the Royal College of Psychiatrists (Robert Kendell) over the role of psychiatry in dealing with 'untreatable' patients. Straw had criticized psychiatrists for not accepting responsibility for these types of 'dangerous and persistent offenders', and for using what he considered to be a 'narrow' interpretation of the law to support their non-involvement. In response, Kendell asked Straw to apologize to psychiatrists for Straw's 'ignorance' of the law, and claimed that Straw was trying to get psychiatrists to his 'dirty work' by demanding that they, rather than the criminal justice system, take on the burden of controlling people with personality disorders. Kendell's position is recorded in a *British Medical Journal* news item:

> Dr Kendell, interviewed on BBC Radio 4's *Today* programme, thought that Mr Straw should apologise. He said that the convicted man, Michael Stone, was not mentally ill but had what Psychiatrists call an antisocial personality disorder. He added 'The law is explicit that people suffering from this condition can only be admitted to hospital for treatment against their wishes if "such treatment is likely to alleviate or prevent a deterioration in their condition". *They cannot be stuck in hospital just to protect the public*'. (Warden, 1998b, p1270, added emphasis)

Jack Straw, however, continued to be very critical of psychiatrists in the media. Announcing in the summer of 1999 the joint consultative document by the Home Office and DoH into the indefinite detaining of 'dangerous people with personality disorder', he once again laid into psychiatrists for what he believed was their undue 'disclaimer' on dealing with this group. He stated (again on BBC Radio 4's *Today* programme on 19th July) that the situation of psychiatrists having refined downwards the number and categories of people who they determined were treatable was rather extraordinary and that this could not continue.

Of course not every doctor or nurse in the psychiatric field has side-stepped this responsibility. Mike Launer, a British consultant psychiatrist, is critical of his colleagues for not inspiring confidence:

> Rarely a week goes by without another schizophrenic being turned away from a psychiatric unit, only to be found either dead in a ditch or guilty of a violent crime. The excuses from the professionals are variable: no beds; the patient refused to co-operate; or, even more worryingly, the patient appeared to be well and not in need of treatment ... I think we as professionals need to work harder to reassure the public. (Launer, 1996)

It is not just the public in general who may be in jeopardy from some mentally disordered people. Members of the psychiatric disciplines can be a very obvious target for attacks by the small minority of those to whom they provide a service:

> [Those] who work professionally with the severely mentally ill or psychologically disturbed can expect to run a peculiar risk of violent behaviour from their clients, past and present. (Blom-Cooper, 1996)

Elizabeth Stanton (1996), a mental health worker, wrote in a newspaper article (entitled 'Nightmare beyond the call of duty') about her experience of dealing professionally with a severely disturbed man. The man, diagnosed as suffering from a personality disorder, tried to kill her at her home and was eventually sent to prison. After his release, however, a number of minor crimes were committed against her property, and she received anonymous and threatening telephone calls, actions she suspected were carried out by this man. Subsequently, the man in question was arrested several times for a series of attacks (some of which were very serious) on other people, none of whom would agree to attend court to support a prosecution. Stanton describes how she and her family continued to live under a reign of terror from this man, with him at various times approaching her son, daughter and grandchildren.

Research design

My empirical study of newspaper accounts of the mentally disordered began in 1994. This was the year in which the report of the inquiry into the killing of Jonathan Zito by Christopher Clunis was presented to the Chairman of the North East Thames and South East Thames Regional Health Authorities (Ritchie et al., 1994). The data presented here cover a five-year period (1994–99). Interim results from the study have been published elsewhere (Morrall, 1998, 1999b).

The specific aims of the study were:

1. to assess whether the discourse of 'moral panic' concerning the dangerousness of the mentally disordered is based on fabrication or reality;
2. to examine the premise, espoused by the psychiatric establishment, that the press are responsible for stimulating a public fear of mentally disordered people living in the community, and that any violence performed by this group is insignificant when compared with that conducted by other sections of society.

There are a number of methodological techniques that can be used to study media accounts of particular topics. Media coverage of an issue can be scrutinized using qualitative research techniques (for example, 'content analysis', 'discourse analysis' or 'thematic analysis') designed to draw out various levels of 'meaning' from the documents. Alternatively, a subject can be assessed using specialist procedures such as 'media impact analysis'. Here, quantitative measurements (for example, the number of times words or phrases associated with the subject occur) and a qualitative computation of the strength of the messages being delivered are combined.

In order to address the aims of the study effectively, and to triangulate data sources, I used a systematic procedure extracted from these techniques. It contained the following five stages:

1. On each day of its publication (Monday to Saturday), a hard
    copy of the British national broad-sheet newspaper, the *Guardian*,
    was reviewed. The electronic archive of the *Daily Telegraph*,
    another British national broad-sheet newspaper, was inspected
    retrospectively. All articles (for example, news items, editorials
    and special features) containing narrative associating a mentally
    disordered person with the killing of another individual or indi-
    viduals were amassed.

2. When a story about a mentally disordered person killing someone
    appeared in the *Guardian*, the search for relevant articles was
    expanded to the hard copies of other broad-sheet and tabloid
    daily (including Sunday) newspapers. These were the *Independent*,
    The Times, the *Sun*, the *Daily Mirror*, the *Daily Express*, the *Daily
    Mail*, the *Daily Star*, the *Daily Telegraph*, *Today* (no longer in produc-
    tion), the *Sunday Times*, the *Observer* and the *Sunday Telegraph*.
    Certain newspapers altered their names slightly during the period
    of the study, for example removing or adding the prefix 'Daily'; I
    have maintained one version of the relevant title throughout.

3. Incidental accounts of murders associated with mentally disor-
    dered people (reported, for example, in radio and television
    broadcasts or in local newspapers) initiated a supplementary
    review of broad-sheet and tabloid newspapers.

4. The content of the reports (where available) of independent
    inquiries into individual homicides by those people who had
    been in the care of the psychiatric services was scrutinized.

5. At the end of the third, fourth and fifth years, the collected news-
    paper accounts were collated and analysed both quantitatively
    (in terms of the number of reported killings, the diagnosis of
    perpetrators and court verdicts) and qualitatively (for an overall
    impression and an identification of textual leitmotivs).

The *Guardian* and the *Daily Telegraph* were, therefore, the primary
data sources. When stories germane to the research aims appeared

in the *Guardian*, they triggered off a wider investigation of the other newspapers. The combined daily (Monday to Saturday) readership of the newspapers evaluated in the study (excluding *Today*) is over 12.5 million, and 1.25 million on a Sunday (National Newspaper Circulation, 1999).

The choice of the *Guardian* was arbitrary. There is a high degree of overlap between the content of newspapers because of the use of centralized dissemination agencies for news. Thus, any newspaper could have been used for the purpose of initiating the extended search. Moreover, the *Guardian* provides as legitimate a reservoir of data as any other newspaper because, as I have discussed above, the traditional differentiation of broad-sheet from tabloid, on the basis of the quality of the journalism or the focus of the narrative, is no longer applicable.

Electronic versions of many newspapers became available during the period of this study, some of which have archives containing every edition published going back several years. Computerized trawling services have been designed to review large collections of these electronic editions. Moreover, a number of newspaper companies have produced their own rudimentary systems for hunting particular stories through the use of 'keywords'. These developments allow social scientists with an interest in studying the presentation of social events in the press far easier access to contemporary and previously published articles, and have made the process of analysis much faster.

The electronic form of the *Daily Telegraph* was chosen, for the purpose of data triangulation, as archive material was obtainable from the date of the beginning of the study (i.e. 1994). It is also a political counterbalance to the *Guardian*, the latter having a left-wing editorial inclination, whereas the former leans to the right. More than 1000 articles were surveyed from this source.

Computerized trawling was not, however, used exclusively because of its inherent inadequacies. For example, the examination of newspapers in this way can produce both 'false negatives' and 'false positives'. That is, a computerized search may result in spurious stories being drawn into the trawl, as well as relevant stories being omitted. Moreover, not all hard-copy articles are reproduced electronically, and vice versa. There may also be a difference in emphasis between electronic and hard-copy versions of the same text because of the form that the typescript takes and the way in which the story and its captions are displayed. For example, a story in the *Electronic Telegraph* (appearing on the 27 July 1995) about a homicide ran with the accentuated headline 'Anger of a mother whose son was "killed by mismanagement and incompetence"'. The following caption (a quote from the mother of the victim) sat below the headline in heavy type but in a smaller-sized font:

> He may not have grown up to be prime minister but he would have grown up to be a decent human being

In the hard copy of the same newspaper, however, it was the quotation that was conspicuous, being given a considerably larger font and much heavier typescript than the headline. Only in the hard-copy version did photographs of the killer, of the mother of the victim and of the victim himself (as a child, alongside his handicapped brother) appear.

Moreover, with computerized trawling, single stories are selected, depending on which keywords are chosen. This means that the significance of juxtaposing such items as 'Love across the woolsack' with 'Racey Lacey' (referred to above) would have been left unrecognized. Furthermore, as Soothill & Grover identify, the researcher may undergo a form of 'sensory deprivation' as a consequence of using only computers for this type of research:

> conducting fieldwork at a keyboard takes one far away from the experience of newspapers. At an earlier stage of technology the use of microfilms and microfiches is one stage removed from seeing, touching and smelling newspapers in the same way as readers experience newspapers. The use of computer searches means that no sensory experience is shared directly with the persons reading newspapers for even the written text looks different. (Soothill & Grover, 1997, p595)

In a study of the impact of journalistic prose, it is, therefore, essential for the researcher to engage in the encounter of reading a newspaper in as similar a way as possible to that of the vast majority of its intended audience. Electronic versions of newspapers will become increasingly popular. However, the millions of newspapers retailed each day in their 'hard' configuration to date considerably outweigh the number read electronically.

Catalogue of killing 1994–99

Approximately 2000 newspapers (hard copy) and over 1000 'electronic' articles were scrutinized during the five years of the study. What follows is the list of homicides associated with mentally disordered people that were reported in those newspapers and articles. The references to 'homicidal madness' from these sources came from statements by the police, adjudication by the courts and the publication of reports from inquiries or inquests. Therefore, the dates given relate not to when the incident occurred but to when the story was published.

In some cases, the original incident and the trial are separated by many years or even decades, but it was reported again as a result of another crime being committed, the original crime finally being brought to court, or the killer being discovered to be back in the community (for example, as part of a programme of rehabilitation). Alternatively, the name of the offender could appear on a list of past killings by the mentally disordered within a story of a killing by another person. There are also cases mentioned in which an individual had been charged but not yet sent for trial.

Furthermore, the 'facts' given here may contain a small number of inaccuracies or omissions with regard to, for example, the diagnosis of the culprit, the sequence of events surrounding the murder or the type of sentence given. Moreover, there may have been judicial appeals whereby the verdict was overturned but this was not reported by the press. There may also be a few appeals still in process at the time of this book's publication or filed afterwards.

The terminology used in this list (for example, with reference to the diagnosis of the culprit or the form of identity given to the victim) has been extracted from the original source. The list presented here is, however, probably not exhaustive because of a degree of researcher error. That is, a small number of murders by the mentally disordered written about in the newspapers and articles analysed may have been overlooked. There were also murder reports appearing in parts of the media other than those examined in this study.

Most of the incidents occurred in Britain (i.e. England, Wales and Scotland). Eight, however, were committed outside Britain (one each in the West Indies, Israel and Germany, and five in the USA). Three of those committed in other countries, however, involved British citizens (as victims). An undetermined number of the perpetrators were not of British origin. In a few of the cases cited, the story is of a continuing court case, the result of which did not get reported.

An unrepresentative number of killings reported by the newspapers belonged to (black) ethnic minority groups. This may be the consequence of the actual number of murders committed by people within these groups being higher than that of the white population. Alternatively, it could be the outcome of an already higher number of black Britons within the psychiatric system – especially the compulsory and secure ('hard end') of it (McKeown & Stowell-Smith, 1998). This in itself may be the result of two trends in British society affecting particularly Afro-Caribbean men: a structural disadvantage that leads to an elevated rate of unemployment and imprisonment, and educational underachievement; and perception of 'Big, Black and Dangerous' amongst the public and professionals.

There were 94 incidents reported in the newspapers during the period of the study, involving 116 killings (that is, some of the incidents involved more than one death). Eight of the killers committed suicide. The most common method of killing was through stabbing or slashing the victim ($n = 44$; 38%). Fourteen (12%) victims were bludgeoned to death with a blunt instrument such as a hammer. Ten people (8.6%) people were strangled or suffocated. Eleven (9.5%) died as a result of being shot, 6 (5.2%) were burnt to death, 5 (4.3%) poisoned, 2 (1.7%) dropped from a height and 2 (1.7%) blown up by a grenade. No mention was made of how 22 (19%) of the victims met their deaths.

Forty-four (47%) of the 94 killers had a primary diagnosis of psychosis (principally schizophrenia) and 18 (19%) of personality disorder (including Munchausen's syndrome and alcoholism). Nine (9.6%) of the killers were described as suffering from depression. A dual diagnosis was attached to seven (7.4%) of the killers, but for 16 (17%) no specific diagnosis was given.

The vast majority of the killers were men ($n = 78$; 83%). The gender of the victim was not mentioned in 32 (27.6%) of the cases.

Where the gender was identified, however, more women ($n = 45$; 38.8%) than men ($n = 39$; 33.6%) had been killed.

Fifty (43%) of those who died were unknown to the killer, whereas 38 (32.8%) were closely related (a present or former spouse or lover, parent, child or sibling of the killer). The number who died who were associates of the killer (neighbours, friends, fellow patients in psychiatric care and prison 'cell-mates') was 24 (20.7%). Four (3.4%) mental health workers were also killed.

The court verdicts in the British cases in which fatalities occurred (where these were known and other than suicide) were: manslaughter with diminished responsibility (44 – two of whom were also found guilty of attempted murder); manslaughter (2); murder (11 – three of whom were also found guilty of other serious offences); unfit to plead (2); not guilty by reason of insanity (7); and infanticide (1). The majority (39) were sent to high-security hospitals indefinitely.

The cases were as follows:

Christopher Clunis (1994): Described as a paranoid schizophrenic with a long psychiatric history, stabbed to death Jonathan Zito.

Paul Medley (1994): Described as a paranoid schizophrenic, was convicted of bludgeoning to death a 79-year-old man after Medley had walked out of a psychiatric hospital.

Andrew Robinson (1995): Diagnosed as a paranoid schizophrenic with a history of aggression and admission to psychiatric care (including a high-security hospital), was convicted of fatally stabbing a 27-year-old female occupational therapist in a mental health unit where he was being compulsorily detained. He had previously been convicted of assault and of carrying a firearm with intent to endanger the life of a woman.

Stephen Laudat (1995): Described as a schizophrenic, had been previously convicted for thefts and robberies, one of which involved a knife, was now convicted of stabbing to death a fellow patient whom he believed to be the gangster Ronnie Kray.

Paul Gordon (1995): Described as a 'former psychiatric patient', was convicted of killing an elderly male stranger as the latter fed pigeons near his home.

Joy Senior (1995): Described as suffering from acute paranoid psychosis and depression, and who believed that she was possessed by the devil, was held to have stabbed her three children to death and then drowned herself.

John Rous (1995): Described as suffering from schizophrenia and a personality disorder, who had a long history of mental illness and of drug and alcohol abuse, was convicted of killing a 22-year-old volunteer worker in the home run by the Cyrenians, where he lived.

Michael Buchanan (1995): Was convicted of attacking a former policeman (who died two days later in hospital) by hitting him with a piece of wood and stamping on his face in an underground car park. Buchanan had approximately 13 previous admissions to psychiatric hospital care over a period of nine years. The killing took place within weeks of his being discharged from the last of these admissions (in 1992).

Erhi Inweh (1995): (diagnosis not mentioned – found not guilty through reason of insanity) Held to have killed a 23-year-old woman who worked for the mental health charity MIND.

Gerald O'Dowd (1995): Described as a paranoid schizophrenic, was convicted of killing his wife by stabbing her through the heart.

Adrian Ng (1995): Described as a schizophrenic, was convicted of killing a woman and her two daughters in the 1980s.

Robert Napper (1995): Described as a psychopath and suffering from paranoid schizophrenia, and with previous convictions for theft and the possession of firearms, was convicted of attacking three women, and killing through stabbing another woman, as well as suffocating her four-year-old daughter.

Luke Warm Luke/Michael Folkes (1995): Described as a schizophrenic with a history of violence and previous psychiatric care, was convicted of killing his girlfriend by stabbing her scores of times with a pair of scissors and by battering her with a fire extinguisher.

Nilesh Gadher (1995): Described as a paranoid schizophrenic, a psychiatric outpatient with previous inpatient admissions, was convicted of killing a woman by driving his car at her in a car park.

Christopher Farrage (1995): Described as a Satanist and suffering from paranoid schizophrenia with a history of psychiatric admissions, and a former pharmacist, was convicted of killing his mother by hitting her with a weight-lifting barbell and repeatedly stabbing her.

Patrick Alesworth (1995): Described as suffering from mental illness for more than 30 years, and as having a personality disorder, was convicted of killing his daughter by bludgeoning her with a hammer and stabbing her. He then committed suicide in the grounds of the psychiatric hospital to which he had been admitted after his trial.

Jason Mitchell (1995): Described as a paranoid schizophrenic and psychopath, who had previously been charged with attempted murder and had other criminal convictions, was convicted of killing his father and two of his father's neighbours.

Alan Boland (1995): Described as a 'discharged mental patient' who suffered from depression and alcoholism, who had allegedly confessed to killing his mother with a hammer, committed suicide whilst on remand in prison.

Robert Viner (1995): Described as a paranoid schizophrenic, died from an overdose of drugs after allegedly killing his mother with an exercise weight.

Stephen Wilkinson (1995): Described as a paranoid schizophrenic, was convicted of entering a school (where he had been a pupil), killing a 12-year-old pupil and stabbing two others.

Shaun Armstrong (1996): Described as a psychopath, who had previous psychiatric inpatient admissions, was convicted of abducting, sexually assaulting, mutilating and killing a three-year-old girl who lived not far from his home.

Unnamed (1996): A woman described as 'having been receiving psychiatric treatment' blew herself up and killed two other members of a church congregation in the German town of Frankfurt with grenades that were strapped to her body.

Anthony Smith (1996): Described as a paranoid schizophrenic, was convicted of stabbing to death his mother and 11-year-old half-brother (both receiving scores of knife wounds) weeks after discharging himself from psychiatric care.

Raymond Sinclair (1996): Described as a paranoid schizophrenic with a history of drug abuse and previous admission to a psychiatric hospital, was convicted of stabbing his mother to death with a vegetable knife.

Robert Satin (1996): Described as being of 'unsound mind', referring to himself as Satan and being obsessed with the occult, was convicted of using a shotgun to kill one person and wound 16 others in 1989.

Anthony Roach (1996): Described as suffering from schizophrenia, was convicted of stabbing to death a 24-year-old woman.

Robin Pask (1996): Described as suffering from psychotic disorders (and at the time of his trial from depression and chronic anxiety), was convicted of killing a female lecturer with a knife whilst attending an Open University course.

Robert Layne (1996): A teenager, who was described as a psychopath and having convictions for robberies and assaults, was convicted of killing his mother by stabbing and battering her, and gouging out her eyes.

Ranjeet Matharu (1996): Described as suffering from depression, was convicted of killing his sister through strangulation in 1987 and, subsequent to his release from a psychiatric hospital, of raping a teenage girl.

Gilbert Steckel (1996): Described as suffering from an acute psychotic illness, was held to have killed his mother by stabbing her. He had in the previous 48 hours twice discharged himself from a psychiatric hospital. He committed suicide by cutting his own throat.

Shahid Iqbal (1996): Described as suffering from a schizoid personality, was convicted of wounding by stabbing nine people in a supermarket and in the vicinity, one of whom later died from his wounds.

Howard Hughes (1996): Described as a paedophile, suffering from a chromosomal abnormality and emotional instability, and having a history of violence, criminal convictions and psychiatric inpatient admissions, was convicted of killing a seven-year-old child.

Martin Mursell (1996): Described as a paranoid schizophrenic, who had a previous history of violence, had served a jail sentence for actual bodily harm to his girlfriend, and had also been previously admitted compulsorily to a psychiatric hospital, was convicted of killing his step-father and stabbing his mother.

Wayne Hutchinson (1996): Described as a paranoid schizophrenic, was convicted of killing two people and attacking three others.

Mathew Hooper (1996): Described as suffering from schizophrenia, with previous inpatient admissions to a psychiatric hospital, and past convictions for stabbing and carrying offensive weapons, was convicted of killing a man through stabbing on Christmas Day.

Albert Goozee (1996): Condemned to hang for murder in 1956, his sentence was commuted to life imprisonment. Having served 15 years in a high-security hospital following a diagnosis of paranoid schizophrenia, he indecently assaulted two young girls.

Emma Gifford (1996): A 22-year-old mother, described as suffering from depression from the age of 13 years, was convicted of killing through suffocation her newly born son.

Karen Fox (1996): Described as (possibly) suffering from Munchausen's syndrome by proxy, was convicted of killing her 20-month-old child by administering large dosages of sodium choride.

Darren Carr (1996): Described as suffering from a psychopathic disorder, a former compulsorily detained psychiatric patient with a history of violence, was convicted of killing a mother and her two children. He had set fire to petrol he had poured around the house he shared with them as a live-in babysitter.

Terry Abraham (1996): Described as suffering from schizophrenia, was convicted of killing his wife, stabbing her 35 times.

Celia Beckett (1996): Described as suffering from severe personality problems, was convicted of killing her four-year-old daughter by administering a noxious substance.

Claire Bosley (1996): Described in police psychiatric evidence as suffering from paranoid depression, committed suicide whilst on remand in prison after being arrested on suspicion of killing her husband.

Michael Brookes (1996): Was convicted of killing a teenage girl by stabbing her over 40 times, strangling her and holding her head in a puddle. He had previously attempted suicide and had been treated in a psychiatric hospital.

Richard Burton (1996): Described as suffering from a severe psychopathic disorder, had a history of psychiatric care and a previous diagnosis of endogenous depression and depressive personality disorder, was convicted of stabbing his landlady to death.

Peter Robak (1997): Described as having a long history of mental illness and believing he was possessed by Satan, in 1991 killed a couple who had befriended him, and their 15-year-old son.

Lisa Whayman (1997): Described as schizophrenic, was convicted of killing her 16-week-old-baby by throwing him off a bridge.

Tolga Kurter (1997): A former inpatient of a psychiatric hospital, was charged with the murder of his neighbour who died from multiple stab wounds.

Hugh Scanlon (1997): Described as suffering from a psychopathic disorder, was convicted of stabbing to death with knives and scissors a 71-year-old man who he believed was propositioning him sexually.

Carolyne Lloyd (1997): Described as suffering from Munchausen's syndrome by proxy, was convicted of killing her four-year-old son by feeding him large quantities of sodium chloride in his drinks.

Robert Jeffrey (1997): Described as suffering from paranoid psychosis, was convicted of killing a man by throwing him from a sixth-floor balcony, and of beating another man to death.

Arthur Jackson (1997): Described as a paranoid schizophrenic, was extradited to Britain from the USA (where he was serving a long-term sentence for stalking and seriously injuring an actress), and was convicted of shooting and killing a man in 1967 during a robbery that Jackson was carrying out.

Mushtaq Khan (1997): He was convicted of shooting two of his sons, killing one, as a consequence of what was described as an 'abnormality of mind'.

Michael Horner (1997): Described as suffering from a paranoid personality disorder and depression, was held to have strangled his wife the day after he was discharged from an acute psychiatric ward. He then committed suicide by hanging.

John Du Pont (1997) A multimillionaire who believed he was the Dalai Lama and that ghosts haunted his property, and described as suffering from paranoid schizophrenia, was convicted of killing the Olympic gold medalist, David Schultz.

Diego Cogolato (1997): Believed himself to be the Messiah, and described as having a serious drug and alcohol problem, as well as suffering from depression, was convicted of stabbing to death his lover, the fashion designer Ossie Clark.

Andrew Cole (1997): Described as having a severe personality disorder, and having been treated for depression, was convicted of stabbing to death his former girlfriend, aged 28 years, and her lover, aged 18.

Wilson Adams (1997):[diagnosis not referred to in the press but described in terms of his mental instability] Charged with killing a British woman (who was unknown to him) on a beach in Antigua by hitting her with a plank and a rock, and slashing her throat with a knife.

James Stemp (1997): Described as a 'disturbed teenager' who had been in the care of a number of special treatment centres having displayed signs of personality disorder, psychosis and drug abuse, at the age of 17 strangled a man to death. He had killed the man after forcing him to drive to an isolated area and then tying him to a tree.

Russell Weston (1998): Described as suffering from paranoid schizophrenia, was charged with shooting and killing two police officers guarding the Capitol building in Washington, USA.

Anthony Joseph (1998): Described as a 'mentally ill resident of a hostel' who believed that he was the son of Christ, murdered a social worker by stabbing her over a hundred times.

Unnamed (1998): Described as suffering from a serious depressive illness and an 'escaped psychiatric inpatient', was charged with the murder through stabbing of a man and the attempted murder of the man's wife in their home.

Doris Walsh (1998): Described as suffering from depression for 20 years, and had previously received inpatient psychiatric care, set fire to her flat and killed her neighbour and his 13-year-old son in 1995.

Colin Crabb (1998): Described as having a background of depression and suicide attempts, and a former psychiatric inpatient with a previous conviction for arson, set fire to his flat and killed his neighbour.

Michael Stone (1998): [awaiting appeal] Described as having a severe personality disorder, was convicted of killing a mother and her six-year-old daughter with a hammer, and of attacking and seriously injuring her nine-year-old daughter. He had a history of violent crime and drug abuse, and had previously received psychiatric outpatient care.

Chay Sibley (1998): Described as suffering from schizophrenia and who believed he was God, was convicted of strangling to death his mother and then mutilating and setting fire to her body.

David Roberts (1998): Described as a schizophrenic, was convicted of stabbing his landlord to death, and later stabbing and bludgeoning with an axe a man who disturbed him whilst Roberts was carrying out a burglary.

Christopher Moffatt (1998): Described as a paranoid schizo-phrenic, was convicted of stabbing a man to death and seriously wounded his wife in their home in a random attack, and then commit-ted suicide in the high-security hospital where he was sent after his trial.

Janice Miller (1998) Described as suffering from severe depres-sion, was convicted of poisoning her seven-year-old twins, and then attempted to commit suicide.

Kenneth McCaskill (1998): Described as a schizophrenic who believed he was Lucifer, was convicted of killing his father and seri-ously wounding his mother with a knife.

Richard Linford (1998): Described as a paranoid schizophrenic with a history of violence, was convicted of killing a man (who also suffered from mental illness) with whom he shared a prison cell.

Wayne Licorish (1998): Described as a schizophrenic with a history of mental problems, was convicted of battering and asphyxi-ating a female stranger.

Desmond Ledgester (1998): Described as a schizophrenic, was convicted of killing his neighbour through strangulation.

Daniel Joseph (1998): Described as psychotic, with a history of violence and a previous psychiatric admission at the age of 17, was at 18 years of age convicted of battering two women, killing one of them.

Peter Horrod (1998): Described as suffering from depression, was convicted of battering with a hammer, suffocating and cutting the throat of his disabled wife.

Justine Cummings (1998): Described as suffering from a psycho-pathic disorder, was convicted of stabbing and thereby killing her boyfriend during a sadomasochistic and drunken sex-game.

Magdi Elgizouli (1998): Described as a paranoid schizophrenic, was convicted of killing a policewoman through stabbing her with a kitchen knife when she and other officers went to arrest him in his bedsit for a breach of bail conditions in connection with an arson attack.

Nicholas Burton (1998): Described as a paranoid schizophrenic, was reported to have admitted to the killing of a woman by slashing her throat.

Michael Carneal (1998): A 15 year-old boy, described as suffer-ing from paranoia and 'schizophrenia-like' symptoms, shot to death three fellow school pupils and injured five others.

Cheryl Adams (1998): Described as suffering from Munchausen's syndrome by proxy, was convicted of smothering and thereby killing her 13-month-old son.

Annette Weston (1998): Described as an alcoholic, was convicted of killing her husband through stabbing him in front of her two children.

Michael Parsonage (1999): Described as suffering from a depressive illness and in a state of 'turmoil' because of a sexual affair he was conducting with a colleague, killed his wife by repeatedly hitting her head with a hammer. Only hours earlier, he had been prescribed tranquillizers by doctors at a local psychiatric crisis unit but had allegedly had his request for further help refused. Parsonage then attempted to commit suicide.

Wayne Tute (1999): Described as a compulsorily detained psychiatric patient who had absconded from hospital whilst on authorized leave, was arrested and charged in connection with the stabbing to death of a man with a steak knife and the attempted murder of a woman.

Louise Sullivan (1999): Described as having a psychopathic disorder and as being on the edges of mental retardation as a result of hypothyroidism, was convicted of shaking to death a six-month-old baby for whom she was employed as a nanny. She returned to her native Australia.

Craig Aaron Smith (1999): Described as 'a very dangerous young man' suffering from 'an emotionally unstable personality', beat, shot with an airgun and strangled a 13-year-old girl.

Jonathan Schmitz (1999): [awaiting retrial] Described as having a history of alcoholism, manic depression and attempts at suicide, was convicted in 1996 of murdering a man three days after the latter had confessed to a homosexual fantasy involving them both whilst they were participating in a television talk-show in the USA.

Kevin Keegan (1999): Described as having a severe antisocial personality disorder with a long history of violence, was convicted of stabbing his wife (whom he had earlier physically abused and threatened to kill) to death on a London street. At the time of the killing, he was on bail for abducting his son-in-law and granddaughter at knife-point.

David Harker (1999): [psychiatric diagnosis not mentioned in the press, but a plea of diminished responsibility accepted by the court] Convicted of killing a mother of four children, and claimed to have eaten parts of her body.

Daniel Okev (1999): A former Israeli soldier, suffering from 'flashbacks' from his undercover work as a member of hit-squads that executed Palestinians, was convicted of killing through shooting a British hitch-hiker in Israel.

Richard Young (1999): Described as suffering from a depressive psychosis, strangled, stabbed and bludgeoned to death with a boulder his wife, whom he believed to be a witch.

Daniel Holden (1999): Described as being seriously mentally ill, kicked and punched his neighbour to death in an argument over a leather coat.

Noel Ruddle (1999): Described as suffering from a severe personality disorder, was in 1992 found guilty of culpable homicide after shooting his neighbour in the Gorbals district of Glasgow. He was given an absolute discharge from a Scottish secure hospital after claiming that, because he was regarded by psychiatrists as being 'untreatable', he could not be legally detained.

Buford Oneal Furrow (1999): Described as having a record of violence and mental illness, and linked to racist groups, was charged with the murder of a man and the attempted murder of five children after opening fire with a gun at a Jewish community centre in Los Angeles.

Unamed (1999): A pensioner (male) was stabbed to death in a random killing on a busy street in Leicester, allegedly by a man who had been discharged from a psychiatric hospital only months previously.

Paul Knight (1999) Described as a paranoid schizophrenic who heard voices telling him to stab black people, he attacked two strangers with a knife, one of whom died of his injuries.

Catalogue of (non-fatal) violence 1994–99

The newspapers also, of course, reported incidents of non-fatal violence and infringements on the lives of others by the mentally disordered. These accounts covered physical attacks on another person, rape, stalking, arson, perceived threats to public safety and wandering around the grounds of a royal residence without an official invitation. All of the incidents occurred in Britain except one (which took place in Canada). The same method adopted to examine cases of homicide in (selected parts of) the media was used to formulate the following catalogue of (non-fatal) violence.

David Morgan (1994): Described as suffering from schizophrenia, hypomania and depressive psychosis, and a psychopath, attacked shoppers and staff (13 women and two men) with a butcher's knife in a department store, and slashed the throat of a nurse with a razor blade whilst on remand in a high-security hospital.

Maria Caseiro (1995): A 29-year-old woman, described as having been released (against the wishes of her consultant psychiatrist) from a mental hospital by a mental health review tribunal, was convicted of causing a general practitioner grievous bodily harm by stabbing him and was sent to a secure hospital without limit of time.

Unnamed (1995): Described as a housewife (diagnosis not given), stabbed a sailor whom she apparently chose at random, and was sent to a psychiatric hospital.

Douglas and Julie Byelong (1996): Described as having (Douglas) paranoid psychosis and (Julie) a history of mental illness, met and married whilst patients in a psychiatric hospital. On honeymoon, they kidnapped a taxi driver (whom they stabbed) and a six-year-old boy, and stabbed and killed a dog.

Clarence Morris (1996): Described variously (as a consequence of differences in expert psychiatric opinion) as suffering from either untreatable psychopathic disorder or paranoid schizophrenia, with dozens of previous convictions involving unlawful sexual intercourse, violence and rape, stalked and threatened to injure a woman over a period of eight months.

Melvin Bennet (1996): Attacked two women with a knife whilst on leave from a psychiatric hospital.

Horrett Campbell (1996): Described as suffering from paranoid schizophrenia, had been previously convicted for possessing an offensive weapon, entered a nursery school playground and attacked with a machete three children (aged between three and four years) and four adults.

Glenn Grant (1996): Described as a paranoid schizophrenic and a psychopath, and previously convicted of two rapes at the age of 15, committed robbery and armed burglary, assaulted a woman at knifepoint, and raped another woman three times, also at knifepoint.

Adamna Fasuyi (1996): Described as a schizophrenic with a history of inpatient and outpatient psychiatric care, repeatedly slashed her 10-year-old daughter with a kitchen knife, four years previously having allegedly tried to strangle her.

André Dallaire (1996): Described as a paranoid schizophrenic with a long history of mental illness, was accused of scaling the perimeter walls of the Canadian Prime Minister's residence, wandering around the grounds and, armed with a knife, breaking into the house in an apparent assassination attempt.

Martin Gidlow (1996): Described as a psychiatric patient and 'a risk to all women', with a previous conviction for robbery and grievous bodily harm to a social worker, went missing from a hostel, whose staff were alleged not to have informed the police until six days after his disappearance.

Noel O'Connor (1996): Charged with assault and making threats to kill, criminal damage, affray and possessing an offensive weapon, went on the rampage in a church during early morning mass. He was found unfit to plead owing to insanity.

Gregory Mellers (1996): Described as suffering from a personality disorder, with previous convictions for attempted robbery and indecent assault, absconded from a medium-secure psychiatric hospital.

Mustapha Mehrez and Glyn Barron-Hastings (1996): Both men attacked a stranger with a knife and hammer shortly after their release from a psychiatric unit, and were sentenced to seven and five years respectively.

David Howell (1996): Described as schizophrenic with a long history of mental illness, and who had previously threatened his mother with a knife, threatened the manager of a supermarket with a knife and was shot dead by police.

Unnamed (1997): Described as a (male) resident of a mental hospital, went for a stroll around the grounds of Buckingham Palace in the early hours of the morning after breaching security systems.

Unnamed (1997): A 15-year-old boy, described as suffering from a conduct disorder and mood swings, admitted to charges of making explosive substances and to possessing a prohibited weapon after setting off a bomb in a biscuit tin on waste ground.

Malcolm Calladine (1997): Described as having had 'mental problems' for over 30 years, a learning disability and a history of violence (including assaults on children and knife attacks), absconded from a psychiatric hospital where he was compulsorily detained, bought a vegetable knife and stabbed a baby (who was unknown to him) in the stomach.

Donald MacLeod (1997): Described as a schizophrenic with a long psychiatric history who believed he was the son of God, slashed a minister with a knife during a church service, and was detained indefinitely in a secure hospital.

Unnamed (1997): A man described as 'under treatment for mental illness', wearing only shorts and covered in white paint, caused thousands of pounds', worth of damage to goods in a supermarket.

Unnamed (1997): Described as 'mentally ill', this man was alleged to have stabbed a policeman twice in the chest.

Unnamed (1997): A 14-year-old teenager, described as having a severe conduct disorder and being a 'very damaged and vulnerable boy' and a 'very serious danger to the public', was convicted of setting fire to a children's home and was ordered by the court to be detained without limit of time.

Robert Buckland (1998): Described as a psychopath, dangerous and disturbed, 18 years old and homeless, embedded a hunting knife into the skull of a 28-year-old female stranger during a train journey.

Unnamed (1998): Described as a psychiatric (male) inpatient, attacked a stranger (a 73-year-old man) with a hammer in a shop.

Unnamed (1998): Described as a violent and disturbed 22-year-old man, and as suffering from Munchausen's syndrome, who had once tried to strangle a nurse. He was reported to be travelling the country trying to gain admission to psychiatric hospitals (whose staff allegedly were unwilling to admit him because of his 'untreatability' and potential for further assaults).

Nicholas Moon (1998): Described as a 'dangerous stalker' and suffering from a personality disorder, had threatened to throw acid in the face of and kill a woman who had ended their relationship. He was sentenced to a three-year probation order by a judge who expressed his regret at the law not allowing for a custodial sentence or sentencing under the Mental Health Act 1983.

Rashid Musa (1999): Described as a psychopath and 'an evil and dangerous man', raped two strangers (a 16-year-old boy and a 40-year-old woman) at knifepoint. An asylum-seeker, he had been recommended for deportation four years earlier by a judge following an attack on a 15-year-old girl and burglary.

Newspaper headlines

Below are examples of the captions used by the newspapers examined in the study to lead stories about mentally disordered people committing violence (fatal and non-fatal):

> Jon's [Zito] Death Will Always Be With Me (*Daily Mail*)
> 'Evil spirits drove me to kill teacher on beach' (*Daily Express*)
> Five years for mother who killed daughter (*Independent*)
> Discharged patient 'killed his mother' (*Guardian*)
> Monster obsessed by Ripper (*Daily Mirror*)
> Landlady killed by psychopath (*Guardian*)
> Girlfriend killed son of bishop in sex game (*Electronic Telegraph*)
> 'Cannibal' Killer Jailed For Life (*Guardian*)
> Released Patient Strangled His Wife (*Electronic Telegraph*)
> Mental Patient Freed to Kill (*Independent*)
> Mum Killed By Psycho (*Daily Mirror*)
> 'Silence Of The Lambs' Maniac Freed To Kill (*Today*)
> Victims' Relatives Brand Community Care A Failure (*The Times*)
> Danger Mental Patients Evade Care (*Sunday Times*)
> A Dreadful Horrific Act (*Daily Mirror*)
> Evil Hammer Killer Guilty (*Sun*)
> Mad Mick The Hammer Man (*Sun*)
> Knife Nut Kills Carer At Hostel (*Sun*)
> Social Worker Stabbed To Death By A Patient (*Daily Mail*)
> Inquiry Call Into Hammer Horror (*Evening Press* – York)
> A Catalogue of Violence (*Yorkshire Evening Post*)
> Hospitals On Alert For Violent Patient (*Northern Echo* – North of England)
> Attacker Back In Hospital (*Herald* – Glasgow)
> Timebomb Who Killed My Dear Little Rosie (*Daily Mail*)

Newspaper Narrative

The following are examples of regular phrases used by journalists (from those newspapers used in the study) concerning the mental condition of the culprit in incidents where a fatality had occurred:

- evil spirits
- severe mental breakdown
- mentally deranged
- freak act of a lunatic
- mental instability
- acting strangely
- hearing voices telling him to 'kill'
- dangerous and unpredictable
- trouble in controlling his temper
- former psychiatric patient
- violent schizophrenic
- a very dangerous man
- very sick young woman
- a mental patient
- extremely aggressive and paranoid
- rampage of 'mindless and horrifying violence'
- paranoid delusions
- behaviour increasingly threatening and violent
- he had a violent psychotic episode, went berserk
- explosive frenzied violence without any obvious provocation
- damaged, mentally unstable
- uncontrollable urge to commit violence
- exceptionally dangerous
- unleashed a hurricane of unmitigated violence
- grandiose ideas
- increasingly mad
- crazed teenager
- frenzied attack
- vicious attack
- a considerable danger to the public
- like living next to a wild uncontrollable animal
- this monster
- suffered from delusions and hallucinations
- a grave anger to the public
- frenzy of stabbing
- hearing voices telling him to kill
- the voices told him what to do
- just went berserk

- a paranoid schizophrenic on the edge of madness
- crazed killer

Recurrent phrases used by the newspapers in their description of the circumstances surrounding the homicide incidents were as follows:

- failures in procedures
- catalogue of errors
- grave errors of judgement
- inexcusable mistakes
- staff failed to act on signs of a deterioration in his condition
- [relatives] had warned he could kill himself or another person
- inadequate care plans and a breakdown in communications
- serious errors by health service professionals
- further tragedies could occur
- illness not taken seriously by staff
- misdiagnosis [of murderer]
- poor standards in patient care
- released from hospital 'by mistake'
- former mental patients were left without supervision
- twice breached his leave conditions, the same evening he was allowed home
- a scandalous lack of co-ordination and care and cycle of neglect
- despite pleas [from parents] he was discharged
- discharged ... against his [the killer's] will
- stopped taking his medication each time he was discharged
- she [mother of killer] spent hours trying to convince social services department that her son was ill
- another tragic failure for Community Care
- mother had appealed for someone to help
- series of errors were made in the care of a mental patient who went on to kill
- clearly psychotic, but discharged himself
- death ... was unnecessary and avoidable
- [the killer has] a history of non-compliance with his medication and absconding from hospital
- poor staff training and little or no risk assessment of patients

- poor communication between agencies
- his [the killer's] family had pleaded for him to be kept under constant supervision, but they were ignored

Radiated victimization

Compared with a list that could have been compiled of all murders (and violence) committed over the five years of this study, the inventory of murder and mutilation registered here may not be considered by some members of the psychiatric establishment to be significant. However, the summation of people affected directly or indirectly by the killers alone runs into thousands, if not millions. In each instance, there is the wasted life of the victim and the dramatically altered life-course of the culprit. The lives of the close family members and friends of each will be displaced to a devastating extent in the short term and quite possibly permanently. Added to this computation of distress is the reshaping, either moderately or severely, of the lives of the victim's and culprit's associates (for example, neighbours, colleagues and other relatives). Furthermore, rumour-mongering and media reporting causes the anguish to ripple through the wider population.

In this sense, as with all murders, it is the 'community' that has been violated. However, distinct from other hazards or dreads, the menace of the 'mad murderer' is construed as being inherently termagant and volatile, a danger that cannot be planned against. Motorcyclists and bicyclists can don crash helmets to guard against head injury, sky-divers can wear an extra parachute in case the first fails to open, and we can devise educational campaigns to reduce the risk of our progeny ingesting illicit drugs or being sexually abused. We could even avoid the potential for injury and death at the hands of a lover or spouse by not indulging in relationships based on emotion. The *crime passionnel*, the root of most murders, is contingent upon a premeditated engagement in interpersonal alliances.

But the possibility of receiving a fatal knife wound inspired by the psychotic or psychopathic proclivities of either a loved one or a complete stranger is regarded as random and indeterminate, and therefore all the more terrifying.

Moreover, unlike 'normal' killings, murders by the mentally disordered are perceived to undermine not only the safety of the citizen, but also the 'rational' basis of the social system. It is the 'madness' of the individual murder, rather than the absolute or relative number of murders by the mad, that generates psychological and social instability. Warranted or not, the unpredictability and incoherence of the mentally disordered killer disturbs both the ontological security of the individual citizen and the normative imputations of the *conscience collective*. Consequently, the killing by those deemed to be mentally disordered is a public issue beyond that of other forms of crime.

Reality's first draft

The newspapers are guilty of sloppy, careless and injudicious journalism in the reporting of mad-murders. Pejorative expressions spatter the narrative and captions of stories covering violent and homicidal incidents involving the mentally disordered. However, the use of 'negative' language in the headline and/or text of the story could be viewed as justified given the nature of the crime. How otherwise could the killing of an innocent person, sometimes by horrendous means, be portrayed?

As I have acknowledged, there may be a number of 'mistakes' in the reporting of events by journalists. Moreover, there are certainly inconsistencies in accounts of the same incident between the various newspapers. For example, one newspaper may state that a murder victim was knifed five times, whereas another will determine the number of stab wounds as three. In the main, however, the core story-line is reported in a similar way across the press.

However, the number of killings recorded by the press falls significantly short of either the larger figure produced by such organizations as the Zito Trust or the smaller figure given by the psychiatric establishment. That is, far from generating a 'moral panic' in terms of raw numbers, there is a considerable under-reporting of homicides by the mentally disordered. For example, in the Zito Trust and Institute of Mental Health Law's (1996) publication *Learning the Lessons*, there are cases registered that have not appeared in the press. The same is true of the on-line file of independent inquiries maintained by David Sheppard, Director of the Institute of Mental Health Law. Using these documents, up to 45% of cases do not get any mention in the newspapers. In addition, although obliged legally to commission independent inquiries, the relevant health authority and/or social service may not do so. Therefore, the overall number of inquiries does not indicate the total number of homicides by the mentally disordered.

What is highlighted repeatedly in the newspaper accounts, however, is the deficient communication between individual mental health practitioners and agencies with regard to discharge from care prior to a murder, and the lack of supervision (particularly over medication). Moreover, attention is drawn to the number of occasions when the person who committed the murder had previously been under the care of the mental health service. It is, therefore, in the interest of the psychiatric disciplines to interpret the reporting of their professional gaffes as media orchestrated 'panics'.

Moreover, it is not a 'media discourse' that is being presented in the headlines and narrative of the newspapers. Journalists are essentially replicating the interpretation of events made by others. Some of the phrases contained in the newspapers are extracted from comments made by those immediately involved with the relevant case (for example, relatives of the victim or killer, the case judge and senior health and social service managers), politicians and representatives of mental health charities and pressure groups. Most of the content, however, originates from the reports of the independent inquiries. That is, nearly all of these descriptions appear in the text of the independent reports, and these reports have been compiled through the collection and triangulation of evidence (given by those connected with the case and expert witnesses, and extracted from germane documents). There is deserved criticism of the 'social process' of an inquiry, and perhaps a need to see a new format evolve in order to increase the validity and reliability of the data supplied and conclusions reached (Peay, 1996), but the information compiled and disseminated through this route is at the very least a realistic approximation of what happened.

Criticism directed towards both practitioners and the health service is more frequent and more prominent in the newspapers than are 'moral panics' about the dangerousness of the mad. That is, it is not the mentally disordered who are being maligned, but those responsible for their care – practitioners, managers of the health service and politicians. If a moral panic were being orchestrated during the 1990s, it was directed at the psychiatric disciplines and systems of mental health care.

Moreover, the editions of the newspapers examined in this study were peppered with alternative commentaries to that of the 'Mad Axeman' type of story. There were articles that discussed the debilitating nature and common incidence of mental disorder and what treatments are available. Other articles offered advice on strategies for reducing stress at work or how to maintain relationships. Pressure groups and voluntary organizations were able to gain space in the newspapers to emphasize the needs of the mentally disordered and the continuing detrimental effects of prejudicial and 'not in my back yard' attitudes. Accounts of suicides, whether or not by people expressly acknowledged as being mentally disordered, are recorded with regularity and usually in a sympathetic vein:

> YOUNG MOTHER KILLED HERSELF: A woman killed herself with a shotgun because she was suffering from post-natal depression ... days after she gave birth prematurely ... Recording a verdict of suicide, [the coroner] said: 'It is clearly difficult even for a woman with post-natal depression to describe how it feels. I only wish the medical profession could do more to help.' (Carter, *Guardian*, 15 May 98)

The newspapers also inform their readers of research that directly challenges the highly stereotypical images that their journalists are accused of perpetuating. For example, various newspapers have recounted the outcome of research into the high number of suicides by mentally disordered people compared with the level of their involvement in homicide. Also appearing in the press are the conclusions from studies into which elements of society the public should most fear. The following headline and narrative, referring to the danger from people under the influence of alcohol and drugs, compared with that posed by mentally disordered people, expressly states the view of the psychiatric establishment:

> MENTALLY ILL 'POSE LESS THREAT THAN ADDICTS': ... the public are more at risk from drunks and people on drugs, psychiatrists said yesterday. There was real evidence that people suffering from mental illness

were no more likely to kill complete strangers than any other groups or individuals. (Hall, *Electronic Telegraph*, 6 January 99)

However, I accept that, compared with the 'sensationalist' reporting of violence by the mentally disordered, the frequency and weight of these counterbalancing inputs is negligible and tends to be consolidated in the broad-sheet portion of the newspaper market.

On the other hand, homicides by 'normal' people are described in a similar fashion to those in which mental disorder is an issue. That is, a mixture of the 'facts' (as provided by the police or through the courts), 'human interest' elements (for example, interviews with relatives and previous associates of the victim or suspect, or witnesses to the crime) and headlines laden with hyperbole is common to both. However, an important difference lies in the way in which the 'mad-murder' is portrayed as 'senseless' and 'motiveless'. Reasons for a 'normal' murder are sought and reported. For example, in the barbaric case in Britain of two students who killed and butchered a close friend (which on the surface seemed inexplicable), the line taken by the judge, and reiterated by the press, was that particular movies watched by the two murderers had led to a brutilization of their thoughts of, and attitude towards, other humans:

> HORROR VIDEOS INSPIRED STUDENT KILLERS: Two students who killed and dismembered their best friend had been so 'desensitised' by horror videos they no longer understood 'the enormity of killing another person', a judge said yesterday. (Gentleman, *Guardian*, 8 May 99)

The absence of an identifiable cause in the 'mad-murder' is, of course, a teleology. The mentally disordered person killing for no 'reason' justifies the diagnosis of madness. Ostensibly 'unintelligible' homicides are frequently reconstructed as 'intelligible' (and therefore liable to 'normal' justice) by both the judiciary and the media through the identification of 'fault' in significant others (parental inadequacy), society (lax gun laws) or the products of the mass entertainment industry (violent films). Alternatively, where neither insanity nor an external influence can be identified, the epithet of 'loner' may applied as a justification of last resort.

The press inevitably under-report the details of homicidal episodes. This happens with all social events simply because of the restrictions of space within newspapers (or indeed any media form). Distortions from abbreviated accounts of any incident written by journalists, unless a consequence of a biased editorial slant, are no more than that which occurs when any individual is trying to filter and retain the myriad pieces of information obtainable from his or her own observations and/or secondary sources. However, when the narrative of newspapers is compared with that appearing in the inquiry reports of homicides by the mentally disordered, much of the most lurid material concerning the killings is omitted. Furthermore, it is rare for the minute contents of the failings and identities of particular staff from the mental health service contained in the inquiry reports to be extrapolated and itemized in a newspaper. That is, an examination of the circumstances of these crimes as reported by the members of the independent inquiries depicts a far more in-depth picture of terror and professional ineptitude than is found in the press.

Summary

The press perpetuate what Mike Hazelton (1993) has described as 'images of disorder'. It is well understood that the media 'edit' and skew the messages they compose by concentrating on particular parts of a story, and through the use of value-laden adjectives and images (Ramon, 1996). There are undoubtedly interpretative processes in the 'construction' of criminality and deviance that need to be acknowledged. For example, in some cases of murder, the offender is labelled 'mentally disordered' only after he or she has entered the judicial system. That is, the categorization of murderous behaviour as 'insanity' may be one of political or legal convenience intended to explain the inexplicable (Prins, 1995), rather than being an accurate representation of those considered to be the 'norm' of the mad population.

But homicides are 'real' in the sense that people have died and others have been incarcerated. Moreover, whether or not the number of homicides by the mentally disordered pales into insignificance when compared with the number of 'normal' murders is beside the point. Subsequent to the death of Jonathan Zito at the hands of Christopher Clunis, scores of people have been killed, many hundreds more have been left bereaved, and still more are in dread of what could happen.

Conclusion

In the 1990s, a 'mad terror' occurred when the public psyche became ruffled by a fear of 'dangerously mad' people. The terror had a degree of reality to it, but became amplified through the exposure in the media of killings perpetrated by the mentally disordered. However, a portion of the blame for the public panic also rests with the psychiatric disciplines for not acknowledging the gravity of Madness and Murder.

Long-term damage has been done to the acceptance by the community of mentally disordered people because of the 'unrealistic' response by the psychiatric disciplines to genuine and understandable (if inflated) fears about the risk posed by the mentally disordered. Moreover, the perceived dangerousness of mad people (whether 'real', amplified or constructed) should have been dealt with earnestly by mental health practitioners in order to assuage an increased level of scapegoating of an already socially excluded group.

There is, however, an elementary tension in the role and functioning of the psychiatric disciplines that gives rise to uncoordinated occupational performance. This I describe as the 'psychiatric paradox'. On the one hand, doctors and nurses are engaged in the monitoring and containment of deviancy (through the supervision of patients' behaviour both in hospital and in the community, the forcible incarceration of patients and the administration of treatment, and the use of mechanical restraint and seclusion). Moreover, as with every occupation, the psychiatric disciplines are impelled to ensure the survival and proliferation of their 'business' and the careers of their members, even when this results in the needs of the 'customer' being inadequately served. On the other hand, psychiatrists and psychiatric nurses declare an investment in the empowerment of their patients, demonstrate a willingness to act as advocates for those in their care, and offer drugs and therapies aimed at psychological rehabilitation. The synchronization and efficient delivery of mental health practice under these conditions is unfeasible.

Protecting rights

Superimposed on the enigima of the psychiatric paradox is the perennial problem of balancing the rights of the mentally disordered, as humans and citizens, with the rights of the rest of the community and the social system as a whole. Throughout the nineteenth century and first half of the twentieth century, legal and psychiatric practice had been imbued with the principle of *parens patriae*, the belief that the state (and agencies of social control) has a 'parental' responsibility towards its citizens (Colaizzi, 1989). Juxtaposed with eugenicism and a conviction that the public required safeguarding was the idea that the mad were vulnerable and in need of protection by the state. *Parens patriae* clearly has a consequence for civil liberties. The parental authority of the state impinges on the citizen's freedom of action to the point of creating debilitation and dependency. The mentally disordered could be (and still can be) involuntarily confined 'for their own good'.

There is a fundamental violation of civil liberty and the sanctity of the human body with the removal of the common-law right to self-determination when treatment is forced – either in hospital or the community – upon those decreed to be of 'unsound mind' (Fennell, 1996). This is particularly the situation when the 'principle of reciprocity' (i.e. matching the loss of civil liberties with adequate care; Eastman, 1994) is not honoured. Moreover, the brutalization of human dignity can be no more violent than when an individual has his or her freedom terminated and is secluded or restrained during his or her internment.

But abuse of the mad has been a phenomenon of pre-asylum care (in which cruelty on the part of the family of the sufferer led in part to the building of 'protective' institutions) and then asylumdom. During the twentieth century, with the mentally disordered being decamped into the community, both structural and personal abuse became rampant. The mentally disordered were (and remain) over-represented in the lowest echelons of the materially impoverished. If not homeless, they resided in the worst areas of the inner cities, where they frequently succumbed to further social incapacitation through the 'dual diagnosis' of madness and substance misuse (Timms & Balazs, 1997). Mentally disordered people were not only susceptible to 'low-level' physical and psychological defilement by the community, but on occasions their ill-treatment reached unbelievably barbaric proportions:

> Five 'cold-hearted and evil' young friends who tortured a schizophrenic teenager to death were given long jail terms yesterday ... The three women and two men imprisoned and beat Angela Pearce, 18, forced her to drink disinfectant and finally strangled her after six days in a Leeds council flat. (Wainwright, 1999)

This accumulation of direct and indirect abuse propels the mentally disordered into a segregated stratum even within the underclass (Morrall, 1999b). The discrepancy between the 'normal' felon being given a life-sentence – which could mean less than 15 years served in prison – and an 'indefinite' verdict for the criminally insane – which could mean for the natural life of the offender (Macalpine & Hunter, 1991) – illustrates how society segregates the mad into a lowly substratum within the criminal justice system as well.

Moreover, the position of the mentally disordered as social outcasts is demonstrated by their expulsion into forms of incarceration other than that of the asylum, where they may receive only minimal mental health care:

> there are many hundreds of men and women remanded in prison for long periods of time, many of whom suffer from longstanding mental disorder, current mental illness, or both. For them effective treatment is an issue of basic human rights. (Fryers et al., 1998, p1026)

Given the degree of indignity suffered by people with what he describes as 'problems with living', Thomas Szasz adopts a radical 'libertarian' position for the role of psychiatry. He argues that psychiatrists should in no instance whatsoever deprive citizens of their liberty 'even if the security of society requires that they engage in such acts' (Szasz, 1993, p798).

There is the potential for the post-liberal mental health and criminal legislation and policies of the new millennium to give too much weight to the 'rights of the community' at the expense of the individual citizen. As Liz Sayce and David Pilgrim have observed, other dilemmas surface when attempting to deal with the issue of preventing, for example, psychopaths from indulging in violence:

> Is it justifiable that someone with mental health problems can be locked up, without trial, for a crime they may commit in the future, yet someone who regularly gets drunk and beats his wife cannot be? (Sayce & Pilgrim, 1998)

One Scottish study of the work of community psychiatric nursing concluded that an 'overprotective' surge as a consequence of a raised awareness of the 'mad terror' was identifiable:

> There has been recent public concern about the needs of people with severe mental health problems in the community and ten CPNs thought that this concern had affected their ability to meet clients' needs, quoting the tendency of CPNs and GPs to overprotect such clients by frequent visiting or having them admitted to hospital. (Lugton et al., 1998, p76)

But claims of 'overprotectiveness' could be viewed as yet another example of defensiveness on behalf of the psychiatric disciplines. The balance between the rights of the individual and those of society became unsymmetrical during the 1990s. The outcry from the public and the media over the care of the mentally disordered, and the danger that the mentally disordered were believed to manifest, was indicative of how there had become a need to readjust those policies and practices which had been inaugurated in the 1960s. Post-liberalism, in both the mental health service and the criminal justice system, is a reflection of a necessary readjustment to the way in which 'antisocial' behaviour is handled in society.

Realist resolution

In the modern world, we are obsessed with risk. Calculations of probability are made about dying from cancer, crashing in an aeroplane as a result of computer failure, contracting a sexually transmitted disease, winning the lottery and living longer by drinking red wine. Professor Anthony Giddens, in his second BBC Reith Lecture in 1999, argued that risk-consciousness is indeed a new phenomenon:

> in the Middle Ages there was no concept of risk. Nor, as far as I have been able to find out, was there in most traditional cultures. The idea of risk appears to have taken hold in the 16th and 17th centuries, and was first coined by Western explorers as they set off on their voyages across the world. (Giddens, 1999, p1)

Allegations that there is a risk of being murdered by a mad person can, therefore, be seen to be merely part of a wider cultural captivation with an ever-expanding range of threats.

However, the possibility that a person suffering from a mental disorder may cause injury to another person predicates mental health law and those aspects of criminal law which relate to psychiatric dysfunction. That is, the incentive for governments to formulate laws directed at the mentally disturbed has always been one of 'control'.

But most risk-assessment techniques have not been established as valid and reliable predictors of violence. What conclusions can be reached about predicting violence with respect to the mentally disordered indicate the complexity of the issue. For example, the MacArthur Community Violence Risk Study in the USA pointed to the heterogeneity of the mentally disordered as a group, as well as to the central role of substance abuse in the prediction of violence amongst people in the community with, and those without, a mental disorder (MacArthur Research Network, 1998).

This does not, however, mean that there cannot ever be measures found that can anticipate dangerousness. Indeed, the MacArthur Research Network on Mental Health and the Law itself has the aim of improving the scientific basis of clinical risk assessment. Professor Herschel Prins provides a 'realistic' evaluation of the status of risk assessment. In answer to the question 'Can dangerousness be predicted?', Prins states:

> If we mean by prediction the capacity to be right every time, the short answer is *no*. If we have more modest goals, should we ask if there are measures, based upon past experience, that could be taken to attempt a possible reduction in dangerous conduct, then the answer is probably *yes*. (Prins, 1995, p230, original emphasis)

Psychiatric medicine and psychiatric nursing must embrace, and be seen to embrace both willingly and effectively, their full responsibilities for the mentally disordered, and extend their commitment to forecasting and dealing with dangerousness to avoid another 'mad terror'.

Psychiatrists and psychiatric nurses have an obligation, both to society and to the mentally disordered, to enact their role as agents of social control. This should over-ride the desire to gain occupational prestige in the market place. The problem of homicides being committed by the mentally disordered must not be ignored simply because the bigger dilemma of what to do about crime by 'normal' people is awaiting resolution. The perceived dangerousness of the mentally disordered does warrant society's intervention to safeguard potential victims and perpetrators.

Mercy & Hammond (1999) offer a cautious but nevertheless positive proposal to the social problem of homicide with their public health perspective. They argue for enhanced mechanisms of 'functional surveillance' at national and local levels to gain more data about the context of violence and homicide, and consequently become better informed about risks and prevention. They argue that there is a need for more information about what the antecedents to homicide are, and, more significantly, about what factors contribute to the absence of violence:

> [the] effects of poverty, unemployment, neighborhood socioeconomic isolation, drug trafficking, the easy availability of guns, and neighborhood safety resources ... we need to better understand what conditions in communities, homes, schools, and families tend to reinforce nonviolent patterns of behavior and other forms of healthy development within various at-risk groups. Much can be learned from the experiences of successful and well-adjusted youths and families who endure adverse circumstances. Just as there are natural forms of resistance to infectious disease within populations, there may be natural forms of resistance to the development of unhealthy behavior within communities and families. (Mercy & Hammond, 1999, p309)

A realist perspective argues for the inclusion of the offender, the public, the state and the victim in the analysis of deviancy and crime. Realism debunks the 'moral panic' thesis, which portrays mental disorder, and the perceived threat from the mentally disturbed, as a media-orchestrated fabrication. Realism, although not ignoring the

social processes that produce epiphenomenal psychiatric constructions, provides a theoretical and policy-making framework through
which the needs of the mentally disordered, the victims and society
are given serious attention.

There is no greater abuse than when a society allows its vulnerable citizens to injure or destroy themselves, or to wound or murder
other innocent people. It is a sign of increasing democratization and
citizen empowerment generally that there is moral indignation
about such issues:

> The critics of risk portray the risk of crime as greatly exaggerated, and the
> public as cultural dupes manipulated by the mass media and the risk control
> industries ... [The] greater public awareness of risk is part and parcel of what
> are essentially progressive and democratic processes throughout the world in
> the late twentieth century. The first is that of environmentalism ... Secondly,
> there is a greater repugnance of violence ... The above two demands are
> subsumed by a more general desire that citizenship should encompass a
> degree of control of the world that surrounds us, from the quality of life in
> the streets of our cities to the accountability of public bodies. (Young, 1999,
> p76)

References and citation index

Abercrombie N, Hill S, Turner BS (1994) The Penguin Dictionary of Sociology. 3rd edn. Harmondsworth: Penguin. p. **118**

Abraham J (1995) Science, Politics and the Pharmaceutical Industry. London: University College of London Press. p. **80**

Aitkenhead D (1998) The washing-machine salesmen of the Third Way are very modern. The Guardian, 18 September. p. **68**

Allsop K (1961) The Bootleggers. London: Hutchinson. p. **103**

American Psychiatric Association (1994) Diagnostic and Statistical Manual of Mental Disorders. 4th edn. Washington, DC: APA. p. **86**

Andrews J (1996) Identifying and providing for the mentally disabled in early modern London. In: Wright D, Digby A (Eds) From Idiocy to Mental Deficiency. London: Routledge, pp 65–92. p. **11**

Andrews J, Briggs A, Porter R, Tucker P, Waddington K (1997) The History of Bethlem. London: Routledge. pp. **26, 33, 36**

Appleby L (1997) National Inquiry into Suicide and Homicide by People with Mental Illness: Progress Report. London: DoH. p. **59**

Appleby L (1999) Safer Services: National Inquiry into Suicide and Homicide by People with Mental Illness. London: DoH. p. **59, 60**

Ash P (1998) Personal computers in forensic psychiatry. Journal of the American Academy of Psychiatry and the Law 26(3): 459–66. p. **23**

Atkinson P (1990) The Ethnographic Imagination: Textual Constructions of Reality. London: Routledge. p. **121**

Axelrod RRM (1984) The Evolution of Cooperation. New York: Basic Books. p. **72**

Bailey WC, Peterson R (1999) Capital punishment, homicide, and deterrence. In Smith MD, Zahn MA (Eds) Homicide: A Sourcebook of Social Research. Thousand Oaks, CA: Sage, pp 257–76. p. **54**

Banerjee S, Bingley W, Murphy E (1995) Deaths of Detained Patients: A Review of Reports to the Mental Health Act Commission. London: Mental Health Foundation. p. **58**

Baudrillard J (1981) For a Critique of the Political Economy of the Sign. St Louis, USA: Telos. p. **125**

Baudrillard J (1983) Simulations. New York: Semiotexte. p. **125**

Baudrillard J (1988) Selected Writings. Stanford: Stanford University Press. p. **125**

Bauman Z (1997) Postmodernity and its Discontents. Cambridge: Polity Press. p. **127**

Beck JC (1995) Forensic psychiatry in Britain. Bulletin of the American Academy of Psychiatry and the Law 23(2): 249–60. p. **22**

Becker HS (1963) Outsiders: Studies in the Sociology of Deviance. Glencoe: Free Press. p. **113, 114**

Becker HS (1974) Labelling theory reconsidered. In Rock P, McIntosh M (Eds) Deviance and Social Control. London: Tavistock, pp 42–53. pp. **113, 115**

Bennett C (1993) In the Blood or in the Head? Guardian, 1 June. p. **78**

Bhaskar R (1986) Scientific Realism and Human Emanicipation. London: Verso. p. **134**

Bhaskar R (1989) Reclaiming Reality: A Critical Inroduction to Contemporary Philosophy. London: Verso. p. **134**

Bhaskar R (1997) A Realist Theory of Science. London: Verso. p. **134**

Bhaskar R (1998) Philosophy and scientific realism. In Archer M, Bhaskar R, Collier A, Lawson T, Norrie A (Eds) Critical Realism: Essential Readings. London: Routledge, pp 16–47. pp. **134, 135**

Blom-Cooper L (1996) Victims of a flawed legal system. Guardian, 21 February. p. **167**

Bloom S (1997) Creating Sanctuary: Toward the Evolution of Sane Societies. London: Routledge. p. **91**

Boseley S (1996) Alarm over suicide rate. Guardian, 16 January. p. **58**

Boseley S (1998a) Medical studies 'rubbish'. Guardian, 24 June. p. **81**

Boseley S (1998b) Bad medicine. Guardian, 22 October. p. **81**

Boyd W (1996) Report of the Confidential Inquiry into Homicides and Suicides by Mentally Ill People. London: Royal College of Psychiatrists. p. **58**

Boyle M (1993) Schizophrenia – a Scientific Delusion. London: Routledge. p. **83**

Brannigan A (1997) Self control, social control and evolutionary psychology: towards an integrated perspective on crime. Canadian Journal of Criminology 39(part 4): 403–31. **71, 148**

Brindle D (1997) Defence budget dwarfed by £32 mental health bill. Guardian, 10 October. p. **19**

Brindle D (1998) Bucolic bliss wins over urban angst. Guardian, 1 July. p. **98**

Britchenell J (1971) Social class, parental social class, and social mobility in psychiatric patients and general population controls. Psychological Medicine 1, 209–21. p. **91**

Busfield J (1996) Men, Women and Madness: Understanding Gender and Mental Disorder. Basingstoke: Macmillan. pp. **13, 15**

Campbell D (1999) Hollywood braced for a savaging. Guardian, 7 June. p. **56**

Carvel J (1998) Citizenship may enter curriculum. Guardian, 1 May. p. **67**

Castle S, Usborne D (1998) Blair's third way leads to New York. Independent, 19 September. p. **66**

Chambliss W (1994) Policing the ghetto underclass: the politics of law and order enforcement. Social Problems 41(2): 177–94. p. **137**

Chaudhary V, Walker M (1996) The petty crime war. Guardian, 21 November. p. **143**

Clare A (1976) Psychiatry in Dissent. London: Tavistock. p. **79**

Clark F (1997) Out of Control. The Advertiser (Adelaide, Australia), 1 November. p. **162**

Clarke J, Layder D (1994) Let's get real: the realist approach in sociology. Sociology Review (November): 6–9. p. **133**

Clinard MB, Meier RF (1995) Sociology of Deviant Behavior. 9th edn. Fort Worth, Texas: Harcourt Brace. pp. **48, 74, 93, 94**

Cloward R, Ohlin L (1960) Delinquency and Opportunity: A Theory of Delinquent Gangs. Chicago: Free Press. p. **103**

Cochran J, Chamlin M, Seth M (1994) Deterence or brutilization?: an impact assessment of Oklahoma's return to capital punishment. Criminology 32: 107–34. p. **54**

Cockerham WC (1996) Sociology of Mental Disorder. 4th edn. Upper Saddle River, New Jersey: Prentice Hall. pp. **6, 10, 16, 19, 27, 91**

Cohen A (1955) Delinquent Boys. London: Free Press. p. **102**

Cohen S (1972) Folk Devils and Moral Panics: The Creation of the Mods and the Rockers. Oxford: Basil Blackwell. pp. **118, 120**

Colaizzi J (1989) Homicidal Insanity 1800–1985. Tuscaloosa, AL: University of Alabama Press. pp. **13, 33, 34, 70, 198**

Colombo A (1997) Understanding Mentally Disordered Offenders. Aldershot: Ashgate. pp. **27, 153**

Conrad P (1981) On Medicalisation of Deviance and Social Control. In Ingleby D (Ed) Critical Psychiatry: The Politics of Mental Health. Harmondsworth: Penguin, pp 102–19. p. **78**

Conrad P, Schneider JW (1980) Deviance and Medicalisation: From Badness to Sickness. St Louis: CV Mosby. p. **82**

Craig T, Bayliss, Klein O, Manning P, Reader L (1995) The Homeless Mentally Ill Initiative: An Evaluation of Four Clinical Teams. London: DoH/Mental Health Foundation. p. **96**

Crawford R (1980) Healthism and the medicalisation of everyday life. International Journal of Health Services 10(3): 365–83. p. **82**

Croall H (1998) Crime and Society in Britain. London: Longman. pp. **8, 105**

Cross R, Jones PA, Card R (1988) Introduction to Criminal Law. 11th edn. London: Butterworths. pp. **37, 51**

Daly M, Wilson M (1999) An evolutionary psychological perspective on homicide. In: Smith MD, Zahn MA (Eds) Homicide: A Sourcebook of Social Research. Thousand Oaks, CA: Sage, pp 58-71. p. **76**

Davies N (1999) Watching the detectives: how the police cheat in fight against crime. Guardian, 18 March. p. **9**

Dawkins R (1989) The Selfish Gene. 2nd edn. Oxford: Oxford University Press. p. **75**

Delanty G (1997) Social Science: Beyond Constructivism and Realism. Buckingham: Open University Press. pp. **68, 136**

Department of Health (1998a) Statistics on In-Patients Detained Under the Mental Health Act 1983. Press release (1998/0553). London: DoH. p. **19**

Department of Health (1998b) Frank Dobson Welcomes New NHS Modernisation Measures: New 'Modernisation Fund' for the NHS. Press release (98/272, 2 July). London: DoH. p. **20**

Department of Health (1998c) Frank Dobson Outlines Third Way For Mental Health. Press release (98/311, 29 July). London: DoH. p. **20**

Department of Health (1998d) Expert Advisor Appointed to Start Review of Mental Health Act. Press release (98/391, 22 September). London: DoH. p. **20**

Department of Health (1998e) Strategy Launched to Modernise the Mental Health Service. Press release (98/0580, 8 December). London: DoH. p. **20**

Department of Health (1998f) New £9 Million Mental Health Unit For Oxfordshire. Press Release (98/224, 5 June). London: DoH. pp. **22, 164**

Department of Health (1998g) Modernising Mental Health Services: Sound, Safe and Supportive. London: DoH. pp. **164, 165**

Department of Health (1999a) Mental Health Act Commission Makes Second National Visit. Press release (1999/0285, 12 May). London: DoH. p. **19**

Department of Health (1999b) Mental Health National Service Frameworks. London: DoH. p. **20**

Department of Health (1999c) Reform of the Mental Health Act 1983. London: DoH. p. **20**

Department of Health (1999d) Saving Lives: Our Healthier Nation. London: Stationery Office. p. **68**

Department of Health and Home Office (1991) Review of Health and Social Services for Mentally Disordered Offenders and Others Requiring Similar Services (the Reed Report). London: DoH. p. **27**

Digby A (1996) Contexts and perspectives. In Wright D, Digby A (Eds) From Idiocy to Mental Deficiency. London: Routledge. p. **11**

Doerner K (1981) Madmen and the Bourgeoisie. Oxford: Blackwell. p. **11**

Duce R, Frean A (1998) Plea for mental help over fantasies of childkilling. The Times, 24 October. p. **40**

Duncan J (1998) England Fans on the Rampage. Guardian, 15 June. p. **100**

Durkheim E (1895/1964) The Division of Labour in Society. New York: Free Press. p. **98**

Durkheim E (1897/1952) Suicide: A Study in Sociology. London: Routledge & Kegan Paul. p. **98**

Eastman N (1994) Mental health law: civil liberties and the principle of reciprocity. British Medical Journal 308: 43–5. p. **198**

Engel M (1996) Papering over the cracks. Guardian, 3 October. p. **157**

Engels F (1845/1969) The Condition of the Working Class in England. St Albans: Granada. p. **106**

Eronen M, Tihonen J, Hakola P (1996) Schizophrenia and homicidal behaviour. Schizophrenia Bulletin 22: 83–9. p. **60**

Esquirol JED (1838) Des Malades Mentales. Paris: Baillière. Translated by Hunt EK (1845) as Mental Maladies: A Treatise on Insanity. Philadelphia: Lea & Blanchard. p. **34**

Exworthy T (1998) Institutions and services in forensic psychiatry. Journal of Forensic Psychiatry 9(2): 395–412. p. **23**

Fallon P (1999) Report of the Committee of Inquiry into the Personality Disorder Unit, Ashworth Special Hospital, Volume 1. London: Stationery Office. pp. **22, 23**

Faris R, Dunham W (1965) Mental Disorders in Urban Areas. Chicago: University of Chicago Press. p. **96**

Fennell P (1996) Treatment Without Consent: Law, Psychiatry and the Treatment of Mentally Disordered People since 1845. London: Routledge. pp. **18, 198**

Fletcher D (1995) Care of mentally ill 'in state of turmoil'. Electronic Telegraph, 25 August. p. **19**

Ford R, Durcan G, Warner L, Hardy P, Muijen M (1998) One day survey by the Mental Health Act Commission of acute psychiatric inpatient wards in England and Wales. British Medical Journal 317: 1279–83. p. **21**

Foucault M (1971) Madness and Civilisation. London: Tavistock. p. **11**

Foucault M (1988) The Dangerous Individual. In Kritzman L (editor) Michel Foucault: Politics, Philosophy, Culture. Routledge: New York, pp 125–51. p. **25**

Fox JA, Levin J (1999) Serial Murder: Popular Myths and Empirical Realities. In: Smith
    MD, Zahn MA (Eds) Homicide: A Sourcebook of Social Research. Thousand Oaks,
    CA: Sage, pp 165–75. p. **52**
Fromm E (1963) The Sane Society. London: Routledge & Kegan Paul. p. **91**
Fryers T, Brugha T, Grounds A, Melzer D (1998) Severe mental illness in prisoners.
    British Medical Journal 317(7165): 1025–6. p. **199**
Garfinkel H (1968) Studies in Ethnomethodology. New York: Prentice Hall. p. **115**
Geddes J, Reynolds S, Streiner D, Szatmari P (1997) Evidence based practice in mental
    health. British Medical Journal 315: 1483–4 (Medline). p. **85**
Gelsthorpe L (1997) Feminism and Criminology. In Maguire M, Morgan R, Reiner R
    (Eds) The Oxford Handbook of Criminology. Oxford: Clarendon Press, pp 511–33.
    p. **108**
Gentleman A (1999) Penal reformers condemn rise in prison suicides. Guardian, 5
    January. pp. **14, 22**
Gibbons DC (1994) Talking about Crime and Criminals. Englewood Cliffs, NJ: Prentice
    Hall. p. **1**
Gibson M (1999) Reading Witchcraft: Stories of Early English Witches. London:
    Routledge. p. **29**
Giddens A (1991) Modernity and self-identity: Self and Society in the Late Modern Age.
    Cambridge: Polity. pp. **5, 108**
Giddens A (1997) Sociology. 3rd edn. Cambridge: Polity Press. p. **101**
Giddens A (1998) The Third Way: The Renewal of Social Democracy. Cambridge:
    Polity Press. p. **67**
Giddens A (1999) Runaway World: Lecture 2. BBC Reith Lectures. Internet site:
    http://news.bbc.co.uk/hi/english/static/events/reith_99/week2.html, pp 1–6.
    p. **201**
Gittings J, Ellison M (1999) Death row links US and China. Guardian, 30 April. pp. **54,
    55**
Glueck S, Glueck E (1950) Unravelling Juvenile Delinquency. New York:
    Commonwealth Fund. p. **149**
Glueck S, Glueck E (1968) Delinquents and Nondelinquents in Perspectives.
    Cambridge: Harvard University Press. p. **149**
Goffman E (1961) Asylums. Harmondsworth: Penguin. p. **115**
Goffman E (1963) Stigma: Notes on the Management of Spoiled Identity.
    Harmondsworth: Penguin. p. **115, 116**
Gomm R (1996) Mental health and inequality. In Heller T, Reynolds J, Gomm R,
    Mustan R, Pattison S (Eds) Mental Health Matters: A Reader. Basingstoke:
    Macmillan/Open University Press, pp 110–20. p. **91**
Goode E (Ed) (1996) Social Deviance. Needham Heights, MA: Allyn & Bacon. pp. **2, 3,
    93, 95, 101, 105**
Goodwin S (1997) Comparative Mental Health Policy. Sage: London. p. **18**
Gottfredson M, Hirschi T (1990) A General Theory of Crime. Stanford, CT: Stanford
    University Press. pp. **3, 4, 148**
Gouldner AW (1971) The Coming Crisis of Western Sociology. London: Heinemann.
    p. **64**
Gove W (Ed) (1980) Labeling Deviant Behaviour. Beverly Hills: Sage. p. **117**
Gramsci A (1971) The Prison Notebooks. New York: International. p. **122**
Griffiths M (1999) Internet addiction: fact or fiction? Psychologist 12(5): 246–50. p. **109**

Gunn J (1998) Forensic psychiatry at a cross-roads. Current Opinion in Psychiatry 11(6): 661–2. p. **22**

Hall C (1996) Inquiries into killing by patients criticised. Electronic Telegraph, 25 October. p. **163**

Hall S (1998a) McVicar's son guilty of Picasso shotgun robbery. Guardian, 22 May. p. **73**

Hall S (1998b) Christie weeps as he denies using steriods. Guardian, 18 June. p. **74**

Hall S, Jefferson T (1976) Resistance Through Rituals: Youth Sub-cultures in Post-war Britain. London: Hutchinson. pp. **120, 121**

Hall S, Critcher C, Jefferson T, Clarke J, Roberts B (1978) Policing the Crisis: Mugging, the State and Law and Order. London: Macmillan. pp. **120, 121, 122, 123, 162**

Hammond WA (1873) Insanity and ts Relation to Crime. New York: Appleton & Co. p. **34**

Harden B (1999) The film that made a serial killer weep. The Guardian, 25 June. p. **56**

Harpending H, Sobus J (1987) Sociopathy as an adaptation. Ethology and Sociobiology 8(3S): 63–72. p. **87**

Hawkins DF (1999) What can we learn from data disaggregation? The case of homicide and African Americans. In Smith MD, Zahn MA (Eds) (1999) Homicide: A Sourcebook of Social Research. Thousand Oaks, CA: Sage, pp 195-210. p. **45**

Hazelton M (1993) The discourse of mental health reform: a critical analysis. Australian Journal of Mental Health Nursing 2(4): 141–54. p. **195**

Hazelton M (1995) Mental health: deinstitutionalization and the problem of citizenship. Australian and New Zealand Journal of Mental Health Nursing 4: 101–12. p. **125**

Hazelton M (1996) Reporting mental health: a discourse analysis of mental health-related news in two Australian newspapers. Paper presented to Australian and New Zealand College of Mental Health Nurses 22nd Annual Conference, Auckland, New Zealand. p. **161**

Health Education Authority (1997) Making Headlines: Mental Health and the National Press. London: HEA. p. **156, 159**

Heginbotham C (1998) UK mental health policy can alter the stigma of mental illness. Lancet 1352(9133): 1052–3. p. **163**

Helman CG (1994) Culture, Health and Illness. 3rd edn. Oxford: Butterworth-Heinemann. p. **99**

Hetherington P (1998) Seeing crime as 'order maintenance'. Guardian, 29 September. p. **143**

Higgins R, Hurst K, Wistow G (1999) Psychiatric Nursing Revisited: The Care Provided for Acute Psychiatric Patients. London: Whurr. pp. **21, 22**

Hirst P, Woolley P (1982) Social Relations and Human Attributes. London: Tavistock. p. **150**

HM Prison Service (1998) Suicides in Prisons – 'More work still to be done says Richard Tilt' [Director General of the Prison Service]. Press release (1N/98). London: HM Prison Service Press Office. p. **14**

Home Office (1990) Provision for Mentally Disordered Offenders (Circular No. 66/90). London: Home Office. p. **27**

Home Office (1996) The Victim's Charter: A Statement of Service for Victims of Crime. London: Home Office Communications Directorate. p. **147**

Home Office (1998a) British Crime Survey: England and Wales (Issue 21/98). London: Home Office Research, Development and Statistics Directorate Crime and Criminal Justice Unit. p. **8**

Home Office (1998b) Criminal Statistics England and Wales 1997 (Cm 4142). London: Home Office Research, Development and Statistics Directorate Crime and Criminal Justice Unit. pp. **49, 57**

Home Office (1998c) New Drug Treatment Scheme For Offenders Starts Today. Press Release (374/98 October). London: Home Office. p. **146**

Home Office (1999) Managing Dangerous People with Severe Personality Disorder: Proposals for Policy Development. London: Home Office. p. **41**

Horton R (1998) A Stab in the Back. Observer, 11 January. p. **80**

Howitt D (1998) Crime: The Media and the Law. Chichester: Wiley. p. **121**

Howlett M (1998) Medication, Non-compliance and Mentally Disordered Offenders: The Role of Non-compliance in Homicide by People with Mental Illness and Proposals for Future Policy. London: The Zito Trust. pp. **60, 154, 160**

Hughes G (1991) Taking crime seriously? A critical analysis of New Left Realism. Sociology Review (November): 18-23. p. **147**

Ingleby D (1982) The social construction of mental illness. In Wright P, Treacher A (Eds) The Problem of Medical Knowledge. Edinburgh: Edinburgh University Press. p. **17**

Jamison KR (1998) Stigma of manic depression: a psychologist's experience. Lancet 352(9133): 1053. p. **116**

Jenkins P (1994) Using Murder: The Social Construction of Serial Homicide. New York: Gruyter. p. **52**

Jenkins R (1998) Jockey 'was stabbed to death by her lover'. The Times, 4 June. p. **46**

Jenkins R, McCullock A, Parker C (1998) Nations for Mental Health: Supporting Governments and Policy Makers. Geneva: WHO. p. **12**

Jones R (Ed) (1985) Mental Health Act Manual. London: Sweet & Maxwell. p. **11**

Jones SG (Ed) (1995) Cybersociety: Computer-mediated Communication and Community. London: Sage. p. **108**

Kiley S (1998) Apartheid killer accuses Botha. The Times, 4 June. p. **46**

Kramer P (1993) Listening to Prozac. London: Fourth Estate. p. **84**

Kraut R, Patterson M, Lundmark V, Kiesler S (1998) Internet paradox: a social technology that reduces social involvement and psychological well-being? American Psychologist 53(9): 1017-31. p. **109**

LaFree G (1999) A summary and review of cross-national comparative studies of homicide. In Smith MD, Zahn MA (Eds) (1999) Homicide: A Sourcebook of Social Research. Thousand Oaks, CA: Sage, pp 125–45. p. **49**

Launer M (1996) Positive thoughts for negative minds. Guardian, 5 June. p. **167**

Laurance J (1998) Bad conduct may have genetic cause. Independent, 6 February. p. **71**

Lawson H, Appignananesi L (Eds) (1989) Dismantling Truth: Reality in the Post-modern World. London: Weidenfeld & Nicolson. p. **134**

Laycock T (1868) Suggestions for rendering medic-mental science available to the better administration of justice and the more effectual prevention of lunacy and crime. Journal of Mental Science XIV(67): 334–45. pp. **13, 37**

Layder D (1994) Understanding Social Theory. London: Sage. pp. **104, 134**

Lea J (1998) Criminology and postmodernity. In Walton P, Young J (Eds) New Criminology Revisited. Basingstoke: Macmillan, pp 163–89. pp. **127, 130**

Lea J, Young J (1984) What is To Be Done about Law and Order? Harmondsworth: Penguin. p. **137**

Le Fanu J (1997) Rise of the Non-disease. Sunday Telegraph, 7 December. p. **79**

Lemert EM (1951) Social Pathology: A Systematic Approach to the Study of Sociopathic Behavior. New York: McGraw-Hill. p. **113**

Lemert EM (1967) Human Deviance, Social Problems and Social Control. New York: Prentice Hall. pp. **114, 115**

Levi M (1997) Violent crime. In Maguire M, Morgan R, Reiner R (Eds) The Oxford Handbook of Criminology. Oxford: Clarendon Press, pp 841–89. pp. **48, 49**

Link B, Cullen FT, Struening E, Shrout PE, Dohrenwend BP (1989) A modified labeling theory approach to mental disorders: an empirical assessment. American Sociological Review 54 (June): 400–23. p. **117**

Littlewood R (1998) Culural variation in the stigmatisation of mental illness. Lancet 353(9133): 1056–7. p. **116**

Lombroso C (1876) *L'Umo Delinquente*. Turin: Fratelli Bocca. p. **70**

Lugton J, McIntosh J, Carney O, Worth A (1998) Assessment of Need For Community Psychiatric Intervention. Research Monograph No. 3. Glasgow: Glasgow Caledonian University. p. **200**

Lukes S (1974) Power: A Radical View. London: Macmillan. p. **104**

Lupton D (1992) Discourse analysis: a new methodology for understanding the ideologies of health and illness. Australian Journal of Public Health 16(2): 145–50. p. **161**

Lyotard JF (1984) The Postmodern Condition. Minneapolis: University of Minnesota. p. **127**

Macalpine I, Hunter R (1991) George III and the Mad-Business. London: Pimlico [first published in 1969 by Allen Lane]. p. **31, 32, 199**

MacArthur Research Network on Mental Health and the Law (1998) The MacAuthur Violence Risk Assessment Study, Executive Summary. Internet site: http://sys.Virginia.EDU/macarthur/violence.html, pp 1–5. p. **201**

McCallum D (1997) Mental health, criminality and the human sciences. In Peterson A, Bunton R (Eds) Foucault, Health and Medicine. London: Routledge, pp 53–73. p. **25**

MacCulloch M, Bailey J (1991) Issues in the provision and evaluation of forensic services. Journal of Forensic Psychiatry 2(3): 247–65. p. **27**

McGuire M, Troisi A (1998) Darwinian Psychiatry. Oxford: Oxford University Press. pp. **71, 86**

Macionis JJ, Plummer K (1997) Sociology: A Global Introduction. Upper Saddle River, NJ: Prentice Hall. p. **103**

McKeown M, Stowell-Smith M (1998) Language, race and forensic psychiatry: some dilemmas for anti-discriminatory practice. In Mason T, Mercer D (Eds) Critical Perspectives in Forensic Care. Basingstoke: Macmillan, pp 188–208. p. **173**

McRobbie A, Thornton S (1995) Rethinking 'moral panic' for multi-mediated social worlds. British Journal of Sociology 46(4): 559–74. pp. **122, 123, 125, 126, 158**

Maden A, Taylor C, Brooke D, Gunn J (1996) Mental Disorder in Remand Prisoners. London: Home Office. p. **14**

Maguire M (1997) Crime statistics, patterns and trends: changing perceptions and their implications. In Maguire M, Morgan R, Reiner R (Eds) The Oxford Handbook of Criminology. Oxford: Clarendon Press, pp. 135–88. p. **8**

Malik K (1998) Darwinian fallacy. Prospect-Magazine, December. Internet site: http://www.propspect-magazine.co.uk/highlights/darwinian_fallacy/index.html, pp 1–9. pp. **71, 88**

Mann CR (1993) Unequal Justice: A Question of Color. Bloomington, IN: Indiana University Press. p. **138**

Marlowe M, Sugarman P (1997) ABC of mental health: disorders of personality. British Medical Journal 315(7101): 176–9. p. **39**

Marshall A (1998) 6,000 expelled for taking guns to school. Independent, 23 May. p. **52**

Mason T, Mercer D (Eds) (1998) Critical Perspectives in Forensic Care. Basingstoke: Macmillan. p. **23**

Mathews R (1993) Squaring up to crime. Sociology Review (February): 26–9. p. **5**

Mathews R (1997) A cultured left hand. New Scientist, 25 October, pp 30–31. pp. **75, 76**

Mathews R (1998) Flukes and flaws. Prospect-Magazine (November): 20–4. p. **85**

Mathews R, Young J (Eds) (1986) Confronting Crime. London: Sage. p. **137**

Matza D (1964) Delinquency and Drift. New York: John Wiley & Sons. p. **102**

Matza D (1969) Becoming Deviant. New York: Prentice Hall. p. **102**

Meadow R (1999) Unnatural sudden infant death. Archives of Disease in Childhood 80: 7–14. p. **50**

Meltzer H, Baljit G, Petticrew M (1994) Surveys of Psychiatric Mobidity in Great Britain. Bulletin No. 1: The Prevalence of Psychiatric Morbidity among Adults aged 16–64 Living in Private Housholds in Great Britain. London: Office of Population Censuses and Surveys. p. **10**

Mercy JA, Hammond WRMD (1999) Combining action and analysis to prevent homicide. In Smith MD, Zahn MA (Eds) Homicide: A Sourcebook of Social Research. Thousand Oaks, CA: Sage, pp 297–310. pp. **49, 202**

Merton RK (1938) Social structure and anomie. American Sociological Review 3 (October): 672–82. pp. **98, 100**

Messner SF, Rosenfeld R (1999) Social structure and homicide: theory and research. In Smith MD, Zahn MA (Eds) Homicide: A Sourcebook of Social Research. Thousand Oaks, CA: Sage, pp 27–41. p. **92**

Mihill C (1997) Computers 'cause social conversation to come unstuck'. Guardian, 16 July. p. **110**

MIND (1997) MIND's Policy on People with Mental Health Problems and the Criminal Justice System. London: MIND. pp. **22, 27, 28/29**

Morgan M, Calnan M, Manning N (1985) Sociological Approaches to Health and Medicine. London: Croom Helm. p. **78**

Morrall PA (1998) Mental Health Nursing and Social Control. London: Whurr. pp. **78, 168**

Morrall PA (1999a) Social exclusion and madness: the complicity of psychiatric medicine and nursing. In Purdy M, Banks D (Eds) Health and Exclusion. London: Routledge. p. **17**

Morrall PA (1999b) Homicides committed by mentally ill people and the role of the psychiatric disciplines. Science, Discourse and Mind 1(1): 1–11. pp. **147, 168, 199**

Morrow R (with Brown DD) (1994) Critical Theory and Methodology. London: Sage. p. **134**

Mossam D, Kapp MB (1998) 'Courtroom whores'? – or why do attorneys call us?: findings from a surver on attorneys' use of mental health experts. Journal of the American Academy of Psychiatry and the Law 26(1): 27–36. p. **14**

Muijen M (1996) Scare in the community: Britain in moral panic. In Heller T, Reynolds

J, Gomm R, Mustan R, Pattison S (Eds) Mental Health Matters: A Reader. Basingstoke: Macmillan/Open University Press, pp 143–55. pp. **163, 164, 165**

Mullin J (1998) Freedom for IRA pair jailed for killing soldiers at funeral. Guardian, 27 November. p. **47**

National Newspaper Circulation (1999) Quoted in the Guardian, 17 May. p. **170**

Nicholson N (1997) Evolutionary psychology: towards a new view of human nature and organisational society. Human Relations 50(9): 1053–78. p. **71**

Norton-Taylor R (1999) Conflict where politicians called the shots. Guardian, 11 June. p. **43**

Nowak M, Sigmund K (1998) Evolution of indirect reciprocity by image scoring. Nature 39: 573–7. p. **73**

Nuland S (1996) An epidemic of scientific discovery. Time (special issue) 148(14): 8–13. p. **80**

Office for National Statistics (1998) Psychiatric Morbidity Among Prisoners in England and Wales. London: Stationery Office. **14, 22**

Palmer A (1983) The Penguin Dictionary of Modern History 1789–1945. 2nd edn. Harmondsworth: Penguin. p. **95**

Peay J (Ed) (1996) Inquiries after Homicide. London: Duckworth. pp. **163, 192**

Peay J (1997) Mentally disordered offenders. In Maguire M, Morgan R, Reiner R (Eds) The Oxford Handbook of Criminology. Oxford: Clarendon Press, pp 661–92. p. **27**

Penrose L (1939) Mental disease and crime: outline for a study of European statistics. British Journal of Medical Psychology 18: 1–15. p. **27**

Pilgrim D, Rogers A (1999) A Sociology of Mental Health and Illness. 2nd edn. Buckingham: Open University Press. p. **153**

Platt T (1996) The politics of law and order. Social Justice 21(3): 3–13. p. **137**

Porter R (1987) A Social History of Madness: Stories of the Insane. London: Weidenfeld & Nicolson. p. **91**

Poulantzas N (1978) State, Power, Socialism. London: New Left. p. **107**

Prins H (1995) Offenders, Deviants or Patients? London: Routledge. pp. **27, 51, 195, 201**

Prior L (1993) The Social Organisation of Mental Illness. London: Sage. p. **116**

Pursehouse M (1991) Looking at the Sun: into the nineties with a tabloid and its readers. Cultural Studies From Birmingham 1: 88–133. p. **158**

Radford T (1998) 'Magic bullet' trial to target brain cancer. Guardian, 22 October. p. **82**

Raine A (1993) The Pychopathology of Crime: Criminal Behavior as a Clinical Disorder. New York: Academic Press. p. **73**

Ramon S (1996) Mental Health in Europe: Ends, Beginnings and Rediscoveries. Basingstoke: Macmillan/MIND. pp. **160, 195**

Ramsbotham D (1998) Barred from mental health care. Mental Health Practice 1(7): 10–11. pp. **14, 22**

Reed J, Baker S (1996) Not Just Sticks and Stones: A Survey of the Stigma, Taboos and Discrimination Experienced by People with Mental Health Problems. London: MIND. p. **124**

Reiner R (1997) Policing and the Police. In Maguire M, Morgan R, Reiner R (Eds) The Oxford Handbook of Criminology. Oxford: Clarendon Press, pp 997–1049. pp. **127, 128**

Repper J, Sayce L, Strong S, Willmot J, Haines M (1997) Tall Stories from the Back Yard (Executive Summary). London: MIND. p. **124**

Riedel M (1999) Sources of homicide data: a review and comparison. In Smith MD, Zahn MA (Eds) (1999) Homicide: A Sourcebook of Social Research. Thousand Oaks, CA: Sage, pp 75–95. p. **48**

Ritchie JH, Dick D, Lingham R (1994) The Report into the Care and Treatment of Christopher Clunis. London: HMSO. p. **168**

Robins LN (1966) Deviant Children Grown Up: A Sociological and Psychiatric Study of Sociopathic Personality. Baltimore: Williams & Wilkins. p. **91**

Robinson DN (1996) Wild Beasts & Idle Humours: The Insanity Defense From Antiquity to the Present. Cambridge, MA: Harvard University Press. pp. **26, 29, 30, 32, 37**

Rock P (1997) Sociological theories of crime. In Maguire M, Morgan R, Reiner R (Eds) The Oxford Handbook of Criminology. Oxford: Clarendon Press, pp 233–55. p. **115**

Rogers A, Pilgrim D, Lacey R (1993) Experiencing Psychiatry: Users' Views of Services. Basingstoke: Macmillan/MIND. p. **22**

Rose S (1997) Lifelines: Biology, Freedom, Determinism. Harmondsworth: Penguin. pp. **75, 77**

Rousseau J (1762, reprinted 1973) The Social Contract. London: Dent. pp. **63, 64**

Rowden R (1998) Fear of Killers. Guardian, 9 March. pp. **165, 166**

Royal College of Psychiatrists (1997) A Manifesto for Mental Health: Rebuilding Mental Health Services for the 21st Century. London: Royal College of Psychiatrists. p. **163**

Sainsbury Centre for Mental Health (1997) Review of the Roles and Training of Mental Health Care Staff. London: Sainsbury Centre for Mental Health. p. **20**

Sainsbury Centre For Mental Health (1998) Acute Problems: A Survey of the Quality of Care in Acute Psychiatric Wards. London: Sainsbury Centre for Mental Health. pp. **19, 21**

Sampson RJ, Laub JH (1993) Crime in the Making: Pathways and Turning Points Through Life. Cambridge: Harvard University Press. p. **149**

Sartorius N (1998) Stigma: what can psychiatrists do about it? Lancet 353(9133): 1058–9. p. **117**

Sayce L (1997) A fair deal: in the public eye, in working life, as citizens. Information leaflet on the campaign 'Respect: time to end discrimination on mental health grounds'. London: MIND. pp. **124, 125**

Sayce L, Pilgrim D (1998) An equitable life. Guardian, 23 September. p. **200**

Scheerer S, Hess H (1997) Social control: a defense and reformulation. In Bergalli R, Sumner C (Eds) Social Control and Political Order: European Perspectives at the End of the Century. London: Sage, pp 95–130. p. **4**

Scheff TJ (1966) Being Mentally Ill: A Sociological Theory. Chicago: Aldine. p. **115**

Scull AT (1993) The Most Solitary of Afflictions: Madness and Society in Britain, 1700–1900. New Haven, CT: Yale University Press. p. **17**

Seedhouse D (1991) Liberating Medicine. Chichester: John Wiley & Sons. p. **79**

Shakespeare T (1997) Social genetics – a polemical issue. British Sociological Association Network (September): 32. p. **74**

Sheldon WA (1949) Varieties of Delinquent Youth. New York: Harper. p. **70**

Shorter E (1997) A History of Psychiatry. New York: John Wiley & Sons. p. **17, 18**

Sims A (1996) Public aspects of schizophrenia. Critical Behaviour and Mental Health (supplement): 85–94. p. **160**

Singer P (1998) Darwin for the left. Prospect (June): 26–30. pp. **71, 72**

Smart C (1976) Women, Crime and Criminology. London: Routledge & Kegan Paul. p. **107**

Smith AD, Beresford D (1998) Few escape tarnish for apartheid era 'crimes against humanity'. Guardian, 30 October. p. **47**

Smith JC, Hogan B (1988) Criminal Law. 6th edn. London: Butterworths. pp. **38, 45**

Smith MD, Zahn MA (Eds) (1999) Homicide: A Sourcebook of Social Research. Thousand Oaks, CA: Sage. p. **9**

Smith PF, Bailey SH (1984) The Modern English Legal System. London: Sweet & Maxwell. p. **28**

Smith RP (1901) A case of epileptic homicide. Journal of Mental Science, XLVII(198): 528–40. p. **35**

Snell T (1997) Capital Punishment 1996 (Bureau of Justice Statistics Bulletin NCJ-167031). Washington, DC: United States Justice Department. p. **54**

Sokal A, Bricmont J (1998) Intellectual Impostures. London: Profile Books. pp. **129, 130**

Soothill K, Grover C (1997) A note on computer searches of newspapers. Sociology 31(3): 591–6. p. **171**

Spinney L (1997) The unselfish gene. New Scientist, 25 October, pp 28–32. p. **75**

Spitzer S (1980) Towards a Marxian theory of deviance. In Kelly DH (Ed) Criminal Behavior: Readings in Criminology. New York: St Martin's Press, pp 175–91. p. **105**

Spungen D (1998) Homicide: The Hidden Truth. A Guide For Professionals. Thousand Oaks, CA: Sage. p. **145**

Stanton E (1996) Nightmare beyond the call of duty. Guardian, 21 February. p. **167**

Stevens A, Price J (1996) Evolutionary Psychiatry: A New Beginning. London: Routledge. pp. **71, 86, 87**

Stone MH (1998) Healing the Mind: A History of Psychiatry from Antiquity to the Present. London: Pimlico. p. **83**

Straw J (1999) New Measures to Protect the Public From Dangerous People. Home Office Press Release (056/99). London: Home Office. p. **40**

Sumner C (1997) Censure, crime and state. In Maguire M, Morgan R, Reiner R (Eds) The Oxford Handbook of Criminology. Oxford: Clarendon Press, pp 499–510. p. **107**

Sutherland EH (1947) Principles of Criminology. Philadelphia: JB Lippincott. p. **148**

Szasz T (1972) The Myth of Mental Illness. St Albans: Paladin.

Szasz T (1973) The Manufacture of Madness. St Albans: Granada. p. **83**

Szasz T (1993) Curing, coercing, and claims-making: a reply to critics. British Journal of Psychiatry 162: 797–800. pp. **16, 42, 199**

Szasz T (1994) Mental illness is still a myth. Society 31(4): 34–9. pp. **12, 16, 127**

Szasz T (1998) Parity for mental illness, disparity for the mental patient. Lancet 352(9135): 1213–15. p. **16, 17**

Taranto N, Bester P, Pierczhniak P, McCallum A, Kennedy H (1998) Medium secure provision in NHS and private hospitals. Journal of Forensic Psychiatry 9(2): 369–78. p. **22**

Taylor I, Walton P, Young J (1981) The New Criminology: For a Social Theory of Deviance. London: Routledge & Kegan Paul. pp. **64, 65, 70, 106**

Taylor PJ, Gunn J (1999) Homicides by people with mental illness: myth and reality. British Journal of Psychiatry 174: 9–14. pp. **60, 154, 155, 163**

Taylor RB and Covington J (1993) Community structural change and fear of crime. Social Problems 40: 374–97. p. **98**

Thames Valley Police (1997) Restorative Justice, Restorative Cautioning – a New Approach. Information leaflet produced by the Restorative Justice Consultancy. Oxford: Thames Valley Police. p. **147**

Thompson K (1998) Moral Panics. London: Routledge. pp. **118, 119, 121, 122, 123**

Thomson JB (1870) The hereditary nature of crime. Journal of Mental Science, XV(72): 487–98. pp. **24, 69**

Thornicroft G (1998) Doing it by halves. Guardian (Society), 11 February. p. **19**

Timms P, Balazs J (1997) ABC of mental health on the margins: mental illness and homelessness. British Medical Journal 315(7107): 536–9. pp. **96, 199**

Traub S, Little C (Eds) (1994) Theories of Deviance. 4th edn. Itasca, IL: Peacock. p. **98**

Tudor K (1996) Mental Health Promotion: Paradigms and Practice. London: Routledge. p. **10**

Unattributed Editorial (1998) The Guardian, 13 January. p. **55**

Waddington PAJ (1986) Mugging as a moral panic: a question of proportion. British Journal of Sociology 37(2): 245–59. p. **123**

Wainwright M (1999) 'Evil' gang tortured teenage girl to death. Guardian, 29 May. p. **199**

Walker M (1998) Clinton and Blair set date for Third Way conference. Guardian, 14 August. p. **67**

Walklate S (1998) Undertanding Criminology: Current Theoretical Debates. Buckingham: Open University Press. pp. **69, 102**

Warden J (1998a) England abandons care in the community for the mentally ill. British Medical Journal 317(7173): 1611. p. **20**

Warden J (1998b) Psychiatrists hit back at home secretary. British Medical Journal 317(7168): 1270. pp. **40, 166**

Waters M (1994) Modern Sociological Theory. London: Sage. pp. **6, 113**

Weatherall D (1995) Science and the Quiet Act: Medical Research and Patient Art. Oxford: Oxford University Press. p. **80**

Webb D, Harris R (Eds) (1999) Mentally Disordered Offenders: Managing People Nobody Owns. London: Routledge. p. **41**

Whitaker R (1998) SA planned chemical war on blacks. Independent, 13 June. p. **46**

Whyte WF (1981) Street Corner Society: The Social Structure of an Italian Slum. 3rd edn. Chicago: University of Chicago Press. p. **121**

Wiglesworth J (1901) Case of murder, the result of pure homicidal impulse. Journal of Mental Science XLVII(197): 335–47. p. **34/35**

Wilczynski A (1997) Child Homicide. London: Greenwich Medical Media. pp. **50, 51**

Wilkins L T (1964) Social Deviance: Social Policy, Action and Research. London: Tavistock. p. **119**

Wolff G, Pathare S, Craig T, Leff J (1996a) Community attitudes to mental illness. British Journal of Psychiatry 168: 183–90. p. **153**

Wolff G, Pathare S, Craig T, Leff J (1996b) Community knowledge of mental illness and reaction to mentally ill people. British Journal of Psychiatry 168: 191–8. p. **153**

World Health Organisation (1999) World Health Report: Global Disease Burden – Leading Causes of Mortality and Burden of Disease, Estimates for 1998. Geneva: WHO. p. **10**

Young J (1986) The failure of criminology: the need for a radical realism. In Mathews R, Young J (Eds) Confronting Crime. London: Sage, pp 4–30. pp. **133, 137, 142**

Young J (1997) Left realist criminology: radical in its analysis, realist in its policy. In Maguire M, Morgan R, Reiner R (Eds) The Oxford Handbook of Criminology. Oxford: Clarendon Press, pp 473–98. pp. **138, 139, 140, 143**

Young J (1998) Writing on the cusp of change: a new criminology for an age of late modernity. In Walton P, Young J (Eds) The New Criminology Revisited, pp 259–95. pp. **139, 140, 141, 143**

Young J (1999) The Exclusive Society. London: Sage. pp. **138, 139, 140, 141, 143, 203**

Young J, Mathews R (1992) Rethinking Criminology: The Realist Debate. London: Sage. pp. **137, 146**

Zahn MA, McCall PL (1999) Trends and patterns of homicide in the 20th century United States. In: Smith MD, Zahn MA (Eds) Homicide: A Sourcebook of Social Research. Thousand Oaks, CA: Sage, pp 9–23. p. **48**

Zedner L (1997) Victims. In Maguire M, Morgan R, Reiner R (Eds) The Oxford Handbook of Criminology. Oxford: Clarendon Press, pp. 577–612. pp. **144, 149**

Zito Trust and Institute of Mental Health Law (1996) Learning the Lessons. 2nd edn. London: Zito Trust, pp 577–612. p. **191**

Zimbardo PG, Bertholf M (1977) Shy murderers. Psychology Today 11(November): 69–70. p. **110**

Zola IK (1972) Medicine as an institution of social control. American Sociological Review 20: 487–504. p. **82**

Subject index